BLACKWELL'S

UNDERGROUND CLINICAL VIGNETTES

EMERGENCY MEDICINE, 2E

BLACKWELL'S

UNDERGROUND CLINICAL VIGNETTES

EMERGENCY MEDICINE, 2E

VIKAS BHUSHAN, MD
University of California, San Francisco, Class of 1991
Series Editor, Diagnostic Radiologist

VISHAL PALL, MBBS
Government Medical College, Chandigarh, India, Class of 1996
Series Editor, U. of Texas, Galveston, Resident in Internal Medicine & Preventive Medicine

TAO LE, MD
University of California, San Francisco, Class of 1996

ROSS BERKELEY, MD
St. Rose Dominican Hospital, Emergency Physician

HOANG NGUYEN, MD, MBA
Northwestern University, Class of 2001

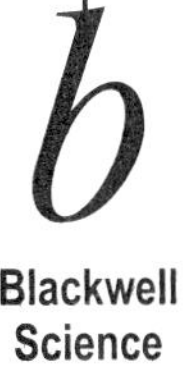

Blackwell
Science

CONTRIBUTORS

Fadi Abou-Nukta, MD
University of Damascus, Syria, Class of 1998

Kalpita Shah, PA-C
University of Texas Medical Branch, Galveston, Class of 2000

Beth Ann Fair, MD
Eastern Virginia Medical School, Resident in Emergency Medicine

Jose Fierro, MBBS
La Salle University, Mexico City

Vipal Soni, MD
UCLA School of Medicine, Class of 1999

Brian Doran, MD
Yale University School of Medicine, Resident in Emergency Medicine

Editorial Offices:
Commerce Place, 350 Main Street, Malden, Massachusetts 02148, USA
Osney Mead, Oxford OX2 0EL, England
25 John Street, London WC1N 2BS, England
23 Ainslie Place, Edinburgh EH3 6AJ, Scotland
54 University Street, Carlton, Victoria 3053, Australia

Other Editorial Offices:
Blackwell Wissenschafts-Verlag GmbH, Kurfürstendamm 57, 10707 Berlin, Germany
Blackwell Science KK, MG Kodenmacho Building, 7-10 Kodenmacho Nihombashi, Chuo-ku, Tokyo 104, Japan
Iowa State University Press, A Blackwell Science Company, 2121 S. State Avenue, Ames, Iowa 50014-8300, USA

Distributors:
The Americas
Blackwell Publishing
c/o AIDC
P.O. Box 20
50 Winter Sport Lane
Williston, VT 05495-0020
(Telephone orders: 800-216-2522; fax orders: 802-864-7626)
Australia
Blackwell Science Pty, Ltd.
54 University Street
Carlton, Victoria 3053
(Telephone orders: 03-9347-0300; fax orders: 03-9349-3016)
Outside The Americas and Australia
Blackwell Science, Ltd.
c/o Marston Book Services, Ltd.
P.O. Box 269
Abingdon
Oxon OX14 4YN
England
(Telephone orders: 44-01235-465500; fax orders: 44-01235-465555)

Acquisitions: Laura DeYoung
Development: Amy Nuttbrock
Production: Lorna Hind and Shawn Girsberger
Manufacturing: Lisa Flanagan
Marketing Manager: Kathleen Mulcahy
Cover design by Leslie Haimes
Interior design by Shawn Girsberger
Typeset by TechBooks
Printed and bound by Capital City Press

Blackwell's Underground Clinical Vignettes: Emergency Medicine, 2e
ISBN 0-632-04561-2

Printed in the United States of America
02 03 04 05 5 4 3 2 1

Library of Congress Cataloging-in-Publication Data
Bhushan, Vikas.
Blackwell's underground clinical vignettes.
Emergency medicine / author, Vikas Bhushan. – 2nd ed.
p. ; cm. – (Underground clinical vignettes) Rev. ed. of: Emergency medicine / Vikas Bhushan ... [et al.]. c1999. ISBN 0-632-04561-2 (pbk.)
1. Emergency medicine – Case studies.
2. Physicians – Licenses – United States – Examinations – Study guides.
[DNLM: 1. Emergencies – Case Report.
2. Emergencies – Problems and Exercises.
3. Emergency Medicine – Case Report. 4. Emergency Medicine – Problems and Exercises. WB 105 B575b 2002] I. Title: Underground clinical vignettes. Emergency medicine. II. Title: Emergency medicine. III. Emergency medicine. IV. Title. V. Series.
RC86.7 .B52 2002
616.02'5'076–dc21

2001004874

Notice

The authors of this volume have taken care that the information contained herein is accurate and compatible with the standards generally accepted at the time of publication. Nevertheless, it is difficult to ensure that all the information given is entirely accurate for all circumstances. The publisher and authors do not guarantee the contents of this book and disclaim any liability, loss, or damage incurred as a consequence, directly or indirectly, of the use and application of any of the contents of this volume.

CONTENTS

MINICASES

MINICASES

ACKNOWLEDGMENTS

Throughout the production of this book, we have had the support of many friends and colleagues. Special thanks to our support team including Anu Gupta, Andrea Fellows, Anastasia Anderson, Srishti Gupta, Mona Pall, Jonathan Kirsch and Chirag Amin. For prior contributions we thank Gianni Le Nguyen, Tarun Mathur, Alex Grimm, Sonia Santos and Elizabeth Sanders.

We have enjoyed working with a world-class international publishing group at Blackwell Science, including Laura DeYoung, Amy Nuttbrock, Lisa Flanagan, Shawn Girsberger, Lorna Hind and Gordon Tibbitts. For help with securing images for the entire series we also thank Lee Martin, Kristopher Jones, Tina Panizzi and Peter Anderson at the University of Alabama, the Armed Forces Institute of Pathology, and many of our fellow Blackwell Science authors.

For submitting comments, corrections, editing, proofreading, and assistance across all of the vignette titles in all editions, we collectively thank:

Tara Adamovich, Carolyn Alexander, Kris Alden, Henry E. Aryan, Lynman Bacolor, Natalie Barteneva, Dean Bartholomew, Debashish Behera, Sumit Bhatia, Sanjay Bindra, Dave Brinton, Julianne Brown, Alexander Brownie, Tamara Callahan, David Canes, Bryan Casey, Aaron Caughey, Hebert Chen, Jonathan Cheng, Arnold Cheung, Arnold Chin, Simion Chiosea, Yoon Cho, Samuel Chung, Gretchen Conant, Vladimir Coric, Christopher Cosgrove, Ronald Cowan, Karekin R. Cunningham, A. Sean Dalley, Rama Dandamudi, Sunit Das, Ryan Armando Dave, John David, Emmanuel de la Cruz, Robert DeMello, Navneet Dhillon, Sharmila Dissanaike, David Donson, Adolf Etchegaray, Alea Eusebio, Priscilla A. Frase, David Frenz, Kristin Gaumer, Yohannes Gebreegziabher, Anil Gehi, Tony George, L.M. Gotanco, Parul Goyal, Alex Grimm, Rajeev Gupta, Ahmad Halim, Sue Hall, David Hasselbacher, Tamra Heimert, Michelle Higley, Dan Hoit, Eric Jackson, Tim Jackson, Sundar Jayaraman, Pei-Ni Jone, Aarchan Joshi, Rajni K. Jutla, Faiyaz Kapadi, Seth Karp, Aaron S. Kesselheim, Sana Khan, Andrew Pin-wei Ko, Francis Kong, Paul Konitzky, Warren S. Krackov, Benjamin H.S. Lau, Ann LaCasce, Connie Lee, Scott Lee, Guillermo Lehmann, Kevin Leung, Paul Levett, Warren Levinson, Eric Ley, Ken Lin,

Pavel Lobanov, J. Mark Maddox, Aram Mardian, Samir Mehta, Gil Melmed, Joe Messina, Robert Mosca, Michael Murphy, Vivek Nandkarni, Siva Naraynan, Carvell Nguyen, Linh Nguyen, Deanna Nobleza, Craig Nodurft, George Noumi, Darin T. Okuda, Adam L. Palance, Paul Pamphrus, Jinha Park, Sonny Patel, Ricardo Pietrobon, Riva L. Rahl, Aashita Randeria, Rachan Reddy, Beatriu Reig, Marilou Reyes, Jeremy Richmon, Tai Roe, Rick Roller, Rajiv Roy, Diego Ruiz, Anthony Russell, Sanjay Sahgal, Urmimala Sarkar, John Schilling, Isabell Schmitt, Daren Schuhmacher, Sonal Shah, Edie Shen, Justin Smith, John Stulak, Lillian Su, Julie Sundaram, Rita Suri, Seth Sweetser, Antonio Talayero, Merita Tan, Mark Tanaka, Eric Taylor, Jess Thompson, Indi Trehan, Raymond Turner, Okafo Uchenna, Eric Uyguanco, Richa Varma, John Wages, Alan Wang, Eunice Wang, Andy Weiss, Amy Williams, Brian Yang, Hany Zaky, Ashraf Zaman and David Zipf.

For generously contributing images to the entire *Underground Clinical Vignette* Step 2 series, we collectively thank the staff at Blackwell Science in Oxford, Boston, and Berlin as well as:

- Alfred Cuschieri, Thomas P.J. Hennessy, Roger M. Greenhalgh, David I. Rowley, Pierce A. Grace (*Clinical Surgery*, © 1996 Blackwell Science), Figures 13.23, 13.35b, 13.51, 15.13, 15.2.
- John Axford (*Medicine*, © 1996 Blackwell Science), Figures f3.10, 2.103a, 2.110b, 3.20a, 3.20b, 3.25b, 3.38a, 5.9Bi, 5.9Bii, 6.41a, 6.41b, 6.74b, 6.74c, 7.78ai, 7.78aii, 7.78b, 8.47b, 9.9e, f3.17, f3.36, f3.37, f5.27, f5.28, f5.45a, f5.48, f5.49a, f5.50, f5.65a, f5.67, f5.68, f8.27a, 10.120b, 11.63b, 11.63c, 11.68a, 11.68b, 11.6c, 12.37a, 12.37b.
- Peter Armstrong, Martin L. Wastie (*Diagnostic Imaging, 4th Edition*, © 1998 Blackwell Science), Figures 2.100, 2.108d, 2.109, 2.11, 2.112, 2.121, 2.122, 2.13, 2.1ba, 2.1bb, 2.36, 2.53, 2.54, 2.69a, 2.71, 2.80a, 2.81b, 2.82, 2.84a, 2.84b, 2.88, 2.89a, 2.89b, 2.90b, 2.94a, 2.94b, 2.96, 2.97, 2.98a, 2.98c, 3.11, 3.19, 3.20, 3.21, 3.22, 3.28, 3.30, 3.34, 3.35b, 3.35c, 3.36, 4.7, 4.8, 4.9, 5.29, 5.33, 5.58, 5.62, 5.63, 5.64, 5.65b, 5.66a, 5.66b, 5.69, 5.71, 5.75, 5.8, 5.9, 6.17a, 6.17b, 6.25, 6.28, 6.29c, 6.30, 7.13, 7.17a, 7.45a, 7.45b, 7.46, 7.50, 7.52, 7.53a, 7.57a, 7.58, 8.7a, 8.7b, 8.7c, 8.86, 8.8a, 8.96, 8.9a, 9.17a, 9.17b, 10.13a, 10.13b, 10.14a, 10.14b, 10.14c, 10.17a, 10.17b, 11.16b, 11.17a, 11.17b, 11.19, 11.23, 11.24, 11.2b, 11.2d, 11.30a, 11.30b, 12.12, 12.15,

12.18, 12.19, 12.3, 12.4, 12.8a, 12.8b, 13.13a, 13.18, 13.18a, 13.20, 13.22a, 13.22b, 13.29, 14.14a, 14.5, 14.6a, 15.25b, 15.29b, 15.31, 15.37, 17.4.

- N.C. Hughes-Jones, S.N. Wickramasinghe (*Lecture Notes On: Haematology, 6th Edition*, © 1996 Blackwell Science), Figures 2.1b, 2.2a, 3.14, 3.8, 4.3, 5.2b, 5.5a, 5.8, 7.1, 7.2, 7.3, 7.5, 8.1, 10.5b, 10.6, 11.1, plate 29, plate 34, plate 44, plate 45, plate 48, plate 5, plate 42.
- Thomas Grumme, Wolfgang Kluge, Konrad Kretzschmar, Andreas Roesler (*Cerebral and Spinal Computed Tomography, 3rd Edition*, © 1998 Blackwell Science), Figures 16.2b, 16.3, 16.6a, 17.1a, 18-1c, 18-5, 41.3c, 41.3d, 44.3, 46.8, 47.7, 48.2, 48.6a, 53.5, 55.2a, 55.2c, 56.2b, 57.1, 61.3a, 61.3b, 63.1a, 64.3a, 65.3c, 66.3b, 67.6, 70.1a, 70.3, 81.2a, 81.4, 82.2, 82.3, 84.6.
- P.R. Patel (*Lecture Notes On: Radiology*, © 1998 Blackwell Science), Figures 2.15, 2.16, 2.25, 2.26, 2.30, 2.31, 2.33, 2.36, 3.11, 3.16, 3.19, 3.4, 3.7, 4.19, 4.20, 4.38, 4.44, 4.45, 4.46, 4.47, 4.49, 4.5, 5.14, 5.6, 6.18, 6.19, 6.20, 6.21, 6.22, 6.31a, 6.31b, 7.18, 7.19, 7.21, 7.22, 7.32, 7.34, 7.41, 7.46a, 7.46b, 7.48, 7.49, 7.9, 8.2, 8.3, 8.4, 8.5, 8.8, 8.9, 9.12, 9.2, 9.3, 9.8, 9.9, 10.11, 10.16, 10.5.
- Ramsay Vallance (*An Atlas of Diagnostic Radiology in Gastroenterology*, © 1999 Blackwell Science), Figures 1.22, 2.57, 2.27, 2.55a, 2.58, 2.59, 2.63, 2.64, 2.65, 3.11, 3.3, 3.37, 3.39, 3.4, 4.6a, 4.8, 4.9, 5.1, 5.29, 5.63, 5.64b, 5.65b, 5.66b, 5.68a, 5.68b, 6.110, 6.15, 6.17, 6.23, 6.29b, 6.30, 6.39, 6.64a, 6.64b, 6.75, 6.78, 6.80, 7.57a, 7.57c, 7.60a, 8.17, 8.48, 8.53, 8.66, 9.11a, 9.15, 9.17, 9.23, 9.24, 9.25, 9.28, 9.30, 9.32a, 9.33, 9.43, 9.45, 9.55b, 9.57, 9.63, 9.64a, 9.64b, 9.64c, 9.66, 10.28, 10.36, 10.44, 10.6.

Please let us know if your name has been missed or misspelled and we will be happy to make the update in the next edition.

PREFACE TO THE 2ND EDITION

We were very pleased with the overwhelmingly positive student feedback for the 1st edition of our *Underground Clinical Vignettes* series. Well over 100,000 copies of the UCV books are in print and have been used by students all over the world.

Over the last two years we have accumulated and incorporated **over a thousand "updates"** and improvements suggested by you, our readers, including:

- many additions of specific boards and wards testable content
- deletions of redundant and overlapping cases
- reordering and reorganization of all cases in both series
- a new master index by case name in each Atlas
- correction of a few factual errors
- diagnosis and treatment updates
- addition of 5–20 new cases in every book
- and the addition of clinical exam photographs within *UCV—Anatomy*

And most important of all, the second edition sets now include two brand new **COLOR ATLAS** supplements, one for each Clinical Vignette series.

- The *UCV–Basic Science Color Atlas* (*Step 1*) includes over 250 color plates, divided into gross pathology, microscopic pathology (histology), hematology, and microbiology (smears).
- The *UCV–Clinical Science Color Atlas* (*Step 2*) has over 125 color plates, including patient images, dermatology, and funduscopy.

Each atlas image is descriptively captioned and linked to its corresponding Step 1 case, Step 2 case, and/or Step 2 MiniCase.

How Atlas Links Work:

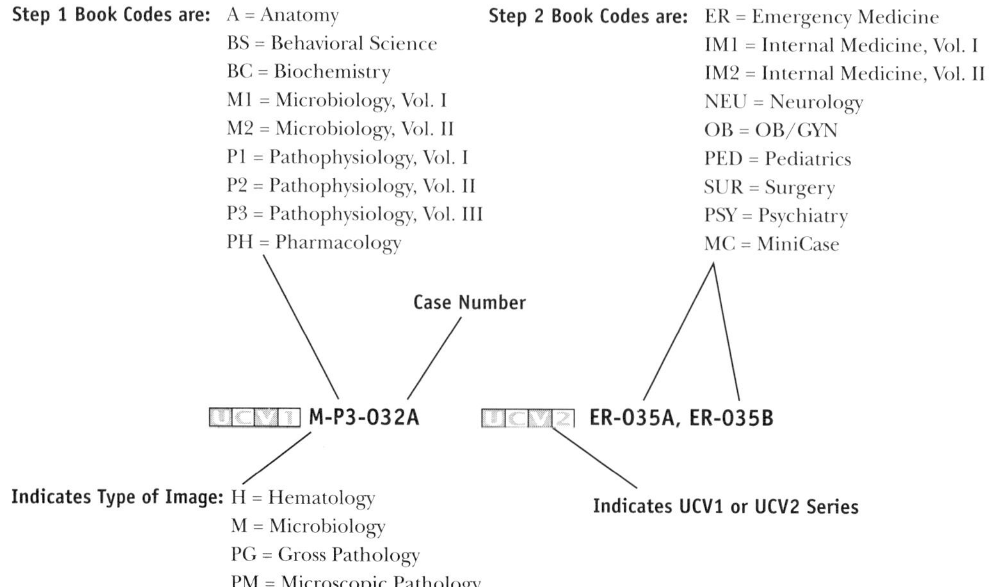

- If the Case number (032, 035, etc.) is not followed by a letter, then there is only one image. Otherwise A, B, C, D indicate up to 4 images.

Bold Faced Links: In order to give you access to the largest number of images possible, we have chosen to cross link the Step 1 and 2 series.

- If the link is bold-faced this indicates that the link is direct (i.e., Step 1 Case with the Basic Science Step 1 Atlas link).
- If the link is not bold-faced this indicates that the link is indirect (Step 1 case with Clinical Science Step 2 Atlas link or vice versa).

We have also implemented a few structural changes upon your request:

- Each current and future edition of our popular *First Aid for the USMLE Step 1* (Appleton & Lange/McGraw-Hill) and *First Aid for the USMLE Step 2* (Appleton & Lange/McGraw-Hill) book will be linked to the corresponding UCV case.
- We eliminated UCV → First Aid links as they frequently become out of date, as the *First Aid* books are revised yearly.

- The Color Atlas is also specially designed for quizzing—captions are descriptive and do not give away the case name directly.

New "MiniCases" replace the previous "Associated Diseases." There are now over **350 unique MiniCases** distributed throughout the ***Step 2 Clinical*** series, selected based on recent USMLE recollections.

We hope the updated UCV series will remain a unique and well-integrated study tool that provides compact clinical correlations to basic science information. They are designed to be easy and fun (comparatively) to read, and helpful for both licensing exams and the wards.

We invite your corrections and suggestions for the fourth edition of these books. For the first submission of each factual correction or new vignette that is selected for inclusion in the fourth edition, you will receive a personal acknowledgement in the revised book. If you submit over 20 high-quality corrections, additions or new vignettes we will also consider **inviting you to become a "Contributor" on the book of your choice**. If you are interested in becoming a potential "Contributor" or "Author" on a future UCV book, or working with our team in developing additional books, please also e-mail us your CV/resume.

We prefer that you submit corrections or suggestions via electronic mail to **UCVteam@yahoo.com**. Please include "Underground Vignettes" as the subject of your message. If you do not have access to e-mail, use the following mailing address: Blackwell Publishing, Attn: UCV Editors, 350 Main Street, Malden, MA 02148, USA.

Vikas Bhushan
Vishal Pall
Tao Le
October 2001

HOW TO USE THIS BOOK

This series was originally developed to address the increasing number of clinical vignette questions on medical examinations, including the USMLE Step 1 and Step 2. It is also designed to supplement and complement the popular *First Aid for the USMLE Step 1* (Appleton & Lange/McGraw Hill) and *First Aid for the USMLE Step 2* (Appleton & Lange/McGraw Hill).

Each UCV 2 book uses a series of approximately 50 **"supra-prototypical" cases as a way to condense testable facts and associations**. The clinical vignettes in this series are designed to give added emphasis to pathogenesis, epidemiology, management and complications. They also contain relevant extensive B/W imaging plates within each book. Additionally, each UCV2 book contains approximately 30 to 60 "MiniCases" that focus on presenting only the key facts for that disease in a tightly edited fashion.

Although each case tends to present all the signs, symptoms, and diagnostic findings for a particular illness, **patients generally will not present with such a "complete" picture either clinically or on a medical examination**. Cases are not meant to simulate a potential real patient or an exam vignette. All the **boldfaced "buzzwords" are for learning purposes** and are not necessarily expected to be found in any one patient with the disease.

Definitions of selected important terms are placed within the vignettes in (SMALL CAPS) in parentheses. Other parenthetical remarks often refer to the pathophysiology or mechanism of disease. The format should also help students learn to present cases succinctly during oral "bullet" presentations on clinical rotations. The cases are meant to serve as a condensed review, not as a primary reference. The information provided in this book has been prepared with a great deal of thought and careful research. This book should not, however, be considered as your sole source of information. Corrections, suggestions and submissions of new cases are encouraged and will be acknowledged and incorporated when appropriate in future editions.

ABBREVIATIONS

5-ASA	5-aminosalicylic acid
ABGs	arterial blood gases
ABVD	adriamycin/bleomycin/vincristine/dacarbazine
ACE	angiotensin-converting enzyme
ACTH	adrenocorticotropic hormone
ADH	antidiuretic hormone
AFP	alpha fetal protein
AI	aortic insufficiency
AIDS	acquired immunodeficiency syndrome
ALL	acute lymphocytic leukemia
ALT	alanine transaminase
AML	acute myelogenous leukemia
ANA	antinuclear antibody
ARDS	adult respiratory distress syndrome
ASD	atrial septal defect
ASO	anti-streptolysin O
AST	aspartate transaminase
AV	arteriovenous
BE	barium enema
BP	blood pressure
BUN	blood urea nitrogen
CAD	coronary artery disease
CALLA	common acute lymphoblastic leukemia antigen
CBC	complete blood count
CHF	congestive heart failure
CK	creatine kinase
CLL	chronic lymphocytic leukemia
CML	chronic myelogenous leukemia
CMV	cytomegalovirus
CNS	central nervous system
COPD	chronic obstructive pulmonary disease
CPK	creatine phosphokinase
CSF	cerebrospinal fluid
CT	computed tomography
CVA	cerebrovascular accident
CXR	chest x-ray
DIC	disseminated intravascular coagulation
DIP	distal interphalangeal
DKA	diabetic ketoacidosis
DM	diabetes mellitus
DTRs	deep tendon reflexes
DVT	deep venous thrombosis

EBV	Epstein–Barr virus
ECG	electrocardiography
Echo	echocardiography
EF	ejection fraction
EGD	esophagogastroduodenoscopy
EMG	electromyography
ERCP	endoscopic retrograde cholangiopancreatography
ESR	erythrocyte sedimentation rate
FEV	forced expiratory volume
FNA	fine needle aspiration
FTA-ABS	fluorescent treponemal antibody absorption
FVC	forced vital capacity
GFR	glomerular filtration rate
GH	growth hormone
GI	gastrointestinal
GM-CSF	granulocyte macrophage colony stimulating factor
GU	genitourinary
HAV	hepatitis A virus
hcG	human chorionic gonadotrophin
HEENT	head, eyes, ears, nose, and throat
HIV	human immunodeficiency virus
HLA	human leukocyte antigen
HPI	history of present illness
HR	heart rate
HRIG	human rabies immune globulin
HS	hereditary spherocytosis
ID/CC	identification and chief complaint
IDDM	insulin-dependent diabetes mellitus
Ig	immunoglobulin
IGF	insulin-like growth factor
IM	intramuscular
JVP	jugular venous pressure
KUB	kidneys/ureter/bladder
LDH	lactate dehydrogenase
LES	lower esophageal sphincter
LFTs	liver function tests
LP	lumbar puncture
LV	left ventricular
LVH	left ventricular hypertrophy
Lytes	electrolytes
MCHC	mean corpuscular hemoglobin concentration
MCV	mean corpuscular volume
MEN	multiple endocrine neoplasia

MGUS	monoclonal gammopathy of undetermined significance
MHC	major histocompatibility complex
MI	myocardial infarction
MOPP	mechlorethamine/vincristine (Oncovorin)/ procarbazine/prednisone
MR	magnetic resonance (imaging)
NHL	non-Hodgkin's lymphoma
NIDDM	non-insulin-dependent diabetes mellitus
NPO	nil per os (nothing by mouth)
NSAID	nonsteroidal anti-inflammatory drug
PA	posteroanterior
PIP	proximal interphalangeal
PBS	peripheral blood smear
PE	physical exam
PFTs	pulmonary function tests
PMI	point of maximal intensity
PMN	polymorphonuclear leukocyte
PT	prothrombin time
PTCA	percutaneous transluminal angioplasty
PTH	parathyroid hormone
PTT	partial thromboplastin time
PUD	peptic ulcer disease
RBC	red blood cell
RPR	rapid plasma reagin
RR	respiratory rate
RS	Reed–Sternberg (cell)
RV	right ventricular
RVH	right ventricular hypertrophy
SBFT	small bowel follow-through
SIADH	syndrome of inappropriate secretion of ADH
SLE	systemic lupus erythematosus
STD	sexually transmitted disease
TFTs	thyroid function tests
tPA	tissue plasminogen activator
TSH	thyroid-stimulating hormone
TIBC	total iron-binding capacity
TIPS	transjugular intrahepatic portosystemic shunt
TPO	thyroid peroxidase
TSH	thyroid-stimulating hormone
TTP	thrombotic thrombocytopenic purpura
UA	urinalysis
UGI	upper GI
US	ultrasound

VDRL	Venereal Disease Research Laboratory
VS	vital signs
VT	ventricular tachycardia
WBC	white blood cell
WPW	Wolff–Parkinson–White (syndrome)
XR	x-ray

ID/CC A **65-year-old male** presents with **sudden-onset, severe, tearing anterior chest pain that radiates to the back**.

HPI He was initially short of breath, anxious, and diaphoretic and then became confused and disoriented. Recently, he noted a dry cough, chest pain, and difficulty swallowing (DYSPHAGIA). He has a heavy **smoking history**, drinks alcohol, leads a sedentary life, and has **hypertension**.

PE VS: **marked hypotension** (BP 60/30) **in right arm**; hypertension (BP 190/120) in left arm; tachycardia (HR 114); tachypnea (RR 35). PE: pale and diaphoretic with central **cyanosis**; hypertensive retinal changes; high-pitched **diastolic decrescendo murmur** (aortic regurgitation due to widening of aortic root); **carotid pulse** asymmetrically **diminished on right side**.

Labs CK-MB and troponin normal. ECG: normal sinus rhythm with left axis deviation and LVH.

Imaging CXR: markedly **widened mediastinum**; cardiomegaly; abnormal aortic silhouette; pleural effusion. Aortogram: evidence of splitting or distortion of the contrast column or of aortic insufficiency is considered diagnostic.

Pathogenesis Associated with **long-standing hypertension** and **cystic medial necrosis** (affecting the ascending aorta, as seen in **Marfan's** and Ehlers–Danlos syndromes). Dissection occurs when blood flowing through an intimal tear splits and flows through muscular layers (dissection is not a true aneurysm). Other causes include trauma, mycotic infection, and syphilis. **Type I** dissections (DEBAKEY) include the proximal (ascending) and distal (descending) aorta; **type II** involve the **ascending** aorta, and **type III** the **descending** aorta. True aneurysms occur most frequently in the abdominal aorta and are associated with **atherosclerosis**.

Epidemiology Aortic dissections occur more frequently in **males** and generally arise in older age groups. Dissection is **more common in the thoracic aorta**. Among untreated patients, the mortality rate is 50% by 48 hours. Patients with bicuspid aortic valve, Turner's syndrome, and coarctation of the aorta are at increased risk. Among young females, 50% of dissections occur during pregnancy.

AORTIC DISSECTION

Management **Hemodynamic stabilization** with fluids and pressors. Subsequently, the patient should receive **nitroprusside and beta-blockers** prior to the initial aortogram. If an ascending dissection is diagnosed, emergent surgery is indicated, as these frequently involve the entire aorta; patients are at risk of developing tamponade, rupture, or acute aortic insufficiency. Dissections requiring emergency resection and replacement with synthetic prosthetic devices are associated with a 15% to 25% intraoperative mortality rate. Uncomplicated, nonprogressive descending aneurysms may be managed medically by controlling BP with nitroprusside and beta-blockers. Evidence of expansion, signs of rupture, poorly controlled BP, or continued pain mandates a thoracotomy.

Complications Complications include dissection into the pericardial sac with cardiac tamponade, stroke, acute aortic regurgitation, MI, rupture with exsanguinating hemorrhage, erosion into vessels with heart failure, embolization, and **sudden death**. "Double-barreled" aorta results if dissection is incomplete.

Atlas Links UCV1 PG-P1-001, PM-P1-001

MINICASE 1: ASYSTOLE

Cardiac standstill characterized by lack of ventricular depolarization and cardiac output

- primary cardiac causes are myocardial ischemia and disease of the SA or AV node, whereas secondary causes include systemic insults resulting in tissue hypoxia or acidosis
- presents with loss of consciousness and unresponsiveness and absent pulse
- flat-line rhythm in 2 perpendicular leads of ECG
- treat with cardiopulmonary resuscitation, epinephrine, and atropine
- complications include permanent neurologic impairment, injury from CPR, and death

MINICASE 2: CAD—PRINZMETAL'S ANGINA

Idiopathic coronary artery spasm

- usually affects women younger than 50 years
- presents with recurrent attacks of severe retrosternal crushing pain occurring at rest
- during the attack, ECG shows ST-segment elevations
- treat with sublingual nitroglycerin for acute pain relief, calcium channel blockers for long-term prophylaxis
- complications include arrhythmia or sudden death

ID/CC A 64-year-old **male** presents to the emergency room complaining of **sudden-onset substernal chest pain** that awakened him from sleep; the pain has lasted for at least 30 minutes.

HPI He describes his pain as a **pressure radiating to the left arm** that is accompanied by mild **shortness of breath, diaphoresis**, and **nausea**. Nitroglycerin only transiently relieved his symptoms, and postural changes and inspiration did not alter his chest pressure. His past medical history is significant for **hypertension and hyperlipidemia**, and his **brother died of an MI at the age of 51**. He additionally reports a 20-pack-year **smoking history**.

PE VS: hypertension (BP 148/68); tachycardia (HR 116); tachypnea (RR 30). PE: obese, pale, and diaphoretic; Sao_2 96% on room air; lungs clear; S_4 gallop noted; no cyanosis or edema.

Labs CBC: normal hematocrit; mild leukocytosis. Lytes: normal. **Elevated troponin T and I; CK-MB levels elevated 4 to 6 hours after pain onset. [A]** ECG: sinus tachycardia; **elevated ST segment** in precordial leads (V_1 through V_6) and leads I and aVL (due to acute anterior wall ischemia), followed by evolving **T-wave inversions and Q waves** occurring in the same lead distribution. (Anteroseptal ischemia produces these changes in leads V_1 to V_3, vs apical or lateral ischemia in leads V_4 to V_6 and inferior wall ischemia in leads II, III, and aVF. Posterior wall ischemia may be indirectly recognized by reciprocal ST depression in leads V_1 to V_3.)

Imaging CXR: borderline cardiomegaly.

Pathogenesis Myocardial infarction is most often caused by a rupture of an atherosclerotic plaque in a coronary artery of the heart, with

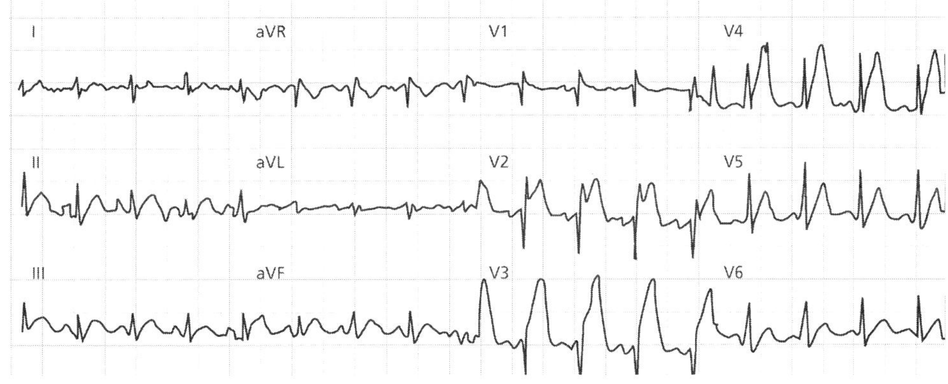

[A]

subsequent thrombosis. The specific location of the coronary artery lesion determines the area of the myocardium affected. Occlusion of the left anterior descending artery results in infarction of the anterior left ventricle and interventricular septum, occlusion of the left circumflex artery causes infarction of the anterolateral left ventricle, and occlusion of the right coronary artery leads to infarction in the posteroinferior right ventricle and interventricular septum.

Epidemiology CAD remains the leading cause of death in the United States. Predisposing factors include **hypertension, cigarette smoking, diabetes, family history, male sex, increasing age**, cocaine use, **dyslipidemia**, and possibly infection with *Chlamydia pneumoniae.*

Management Standard management includes **oxygen, aspirin, pain relief** (usually **morphine sulfate**), and a **beta-blocker** (unless contraindicated). Admit to a coronary care unit; **continuous ECG** monitoring; give sublingual **nitroglycerin** until pain free. Consider nitroglycerin drip; consider **heparin** bolus. The acute treatment is aimed at restoring blood flow to the ischemic region as soon as possible. This is accomplished by emergent catheterization with **balloon angioplasty** (if immediately available) or intravenous **thrombolytic infusion** (unless contraindicated).

Complications **Arrhythmias** (most common cause of death in early post-MI period; usually ventricular fibrillation), pulmonary edema, heart failure, ventricular aneurysm formation, cardiogenic shock, mitral insufficiency, mural thrombosis and embolism, pericarditis (3 to 5 days post-MI), ventricular wall or papillary muscle rupture (5 to 10 days post-MI), and post-MI autoimmune pericarditis (DRESSLER'S SYNDROME) (occurs in 5% of patients at 1 to 12 weeks post-MI; may be recurrent).

Atlas Links UCV1 PG-P1-007, PM-P1-007

MINICASE 3: CAD—UNSTABLE ANGINA

Cardiac ischemic chest pain occurring at rest or showing an increase from typical angina patterns

- ECG shows ST-segment depression and T-wave flattening
- treat with urgent heparinization and coronary angioplasty
- complications include a high risk of subsequent myocardial infarction

ID/CC A 32-year-old firefighter presents with multiple injuries after an explosion. He is **gasping for air** and complaining of severe **light-headedness** and weakness.

HPI During the explosion, a piece of wood **pierced his thoracic wall** at the fifth intercostal space along the left sternal border.

PE VS: tachycardia (HR 130); **hypotension** (BP 90/80) **unresponsive to rehydration** (note the narrow pulse pressure); tachypnea. PE: cyanosis; confusion and acute distress; JVD; **heart sounds distant**; apical impulse diminished; **inspiratory lowering of systolic BP of > 10 mmHg** (PULSUS PARADOXUS); increased distention of neck veins during inspiration (KUSSMAUL'S SIGN).

Labs ECG: nonspecific ST-segment and T-wave changes; diminished QRS voltage in limb leads; QRS complexes alternating in size (ELECTRICAL ALTERNANS).

Imaging CXR: mild cardiomegaly (in acute hemopericardium, the heart may not appear enlarged; thus, diagnosis and treatment are clinical). Echo: accumulation of fluid in the pericardial sac with compression of all chambers; RA and RV diastolic collapse; swinging of the heart; increase in LV dimensions during inspiration; diastolic increase in RV dimensions.

Pathogenesis Tamponade arises when a pericardial effusion develops rapidly or is large enough to compress the heart, impairing venous return, heart filling, and arterial outflow. This may lead to **hypotension, distant heart sounds, and JVD** (BECK'S TRIAD). Cardiac tamponade arises in the context of trauma, heart and lung tumors, ventricular wall rupture during MI, pericarditis, uremia, iatrogenic cardiac rupture during catheterization or pacemaker placement, and rupture of a syphilitic aneurysm of the intrapericardial aorta.

Epidemiology **Penetrating trauma** and automobile accidents (steering wheel blunt trauma) account for a large proportion of cases. Knife wounds tend to seal and produce tamponade, whereas gunshot wound orifices are large and preclude compression.

Management Immediate **pericardiocentesis. IV fluids and pressors** for hemodynamic stabilization. All patients with positive pericardiocentesis due to trauma should undergo exploratory thoracotomy.

Complications Death.

CARDIAC TAMPONADE

ID/CC An **elderly** male is found lying in the street.

HPI The patient is **homeless, abuses alcohol**, and is **mentally ill**.

PE VS: hypothermia (30°C); bradycardia (HR 40); hypotension (BP 90 by palpation); pulse oximeter will not register due to **decreased peripheral perfusion**. PE: unarousable with no signs of trauma; pupils symmetric and sluggish; chest clear with **slowed respirations; decreased bowel sounds**; extremity pulses absent; skin **cold; absence of shivering**; peripheral **cyanosis and frostbite**; depressed cough and gag reflexes and **diminished DTRs**.

Labs Laboratory tests should be performed to **identify any underlying or contributing causes** of the patient's hypothermia. Complete evaluation should include CBC, blood cultures, electrolytes, glucose, ABGs, LFTs, toxicology screen, and UA. TFTs and cortisol levels may be sent as well. **Do not correct ABG results** for hypothermia because "normal" values for these patients are not known. **ECG** may demonstrate the **Osborne wave (J wave)**, a positive deflection seen at the junction of the QRS and ST segments, and low voltage.

Imaging CT, head: may be useful to rule out intracranial hemorrhage and cerebrovascular accident or in patients whose mental status does not improve appropriately with rewarming. Other diagnostic imaging (e.g., x-rays of the cervical spine, pelvis, and chest) should be considered if there is suspicion of trauma. CXR may also reveal evidence of pneumonia or aspiration.

Pathogenesis Hypothermia is defined **as a core body temperature of < 35°C**. It is a clinical state in which the body is unable to generate sufficient heat to function normally. All of the body's organ systems are affected, and there is generalized slowing of all metabolic activity. **Exposure to cold or immersion in cold water** are the primary causes of accidental hypothermia. Other causes include **metabolic** derangements, **drugs, sepsis**, and **CNS dysfunction**. In **mild hypothermia (32.2°C to 35°C)**, the body attempts to retain and generate heat. This phase is characterized by excitation, shivering, tachycardia, and hypertension. With **moderate hypothermia (30°C to 35°C)**, heart rate, cardiac output, and blood pressure are decreased. **Severe hypothermia occurs at temperatures < 30°C**. At this level, the heart is prone to dangerous **arrhythmias**.

Epidemiology Approximately 800 deaths due to hypothermia occur in the United States each year. Individuals at the extremes of age are at particular risk. Alcoholic, mentally ill, and debilitated patients are also at increased risk.

Management Management is based on the level of hypothermia and on the patient's cardiovascular stability. **CPR** should be administered to any unmonitored patient who is severely hypothermic and appears to be in cardiac arrest. Resuscitation should continue until the patient's body temperature is normalized. The patient is not dead until he or she is **"warm and dead."** Cardiac rhythms other than ventricular fibrillation and asystole should not be treated, because they will generally resolve with rewarming. **Bretylium** is the drug of choice for ventricular fibrillation. Gradual, **passive rewarming** is indicated for **mild hypothermia**, including removal from cold and **insulation with warm blankets**. **Moderate or severe hypothermia** requires **active rewarming** by exposing the patient to an exogenous heat source. **Active external rewarming** includes warming blankets, heat lamps, and hot water bottles. **Active core rewarming** includes **warmed IV fluids, warm fluid peritoneal lavage, and warm humidified oxygen. Extracorporeal rewarming** should be considered for severe hypothermia; these measures include **hemodialysis** and **cardiopulmonary bypass. Prophylactic antibiotics** and stress-dose **steroids** should be given based on clinical suspicion. Empiric thiamine, naloxone, and glucose should be given for altered mental status. **Diuresis** due to vasoconstriction and a blunted response to ADH may result in **"rewarming shock."** Moderately to severely hypothermic patients should be admitted to the ICU.

Complications Complications include **death** from **failure to diagnose early** and initiate therapy. The **underlying cause** of hypothermia must be identified. Hypothermic patients are also at risk of developing **rhabdomyolysis**.

ID/CC A **38-year-old male** presents with **severe headache** and **transient blindness**.

HPI He **vomited** but denies any **changes in mental status** or **paralysis**.

PE VS: no fever; **hypertension (BP 220/145)**. PE: alert and oriented ×3; visual fields normal; **papilledema, retinal hemorrhages, and exudates; rales bilaterally in lungs**; S_3 present.

Labs PBS: **schistocytes (microangiopathic hemolysis). Elevated BUN** (60 mg/dL) **and creatinine** (3.5 mg/dL); elevated uric acid (12 mg/dL). **UA: 3+ protein and RBCs**.

Pathogenesis This condition is associated with dilated cerebral arteries and **arteriolar fibrinoid necrosis**. Normal cerebrovascular autoregulation is disturbed as a result of barotrauma, causing excessive flow and consequent encephalopathy. Patients also demonstrate evidence of microangiopathic hemolytic anemia and elevated renin and aldosterone.

Epidemiology Malignant hypertension arises in approximately **1% of hypertensive patients** and occurs more commonly in **men**. The **mean age at presentation is 40**. When untreated, most patients die of renal failure, CHF, or cerebrovascular accidents within 3 to 6 months.

Management Lower BP acutely **by one-third** but not below 160/95 owing to the risk of precipitating watershed infarcts. **Nitroprusside** is the preferred drug, but trimethaphan, nitroglycerin, labetalol, enalapril, diazoxide, and hydralazine may also be used. Loop diuretics are especially useful in cases where pulmonary edema is present. All patients require hospital admission to a monitored bed. Patients should be initiated on long-term antihypertensive therapy, since malignant hypertension is uncommon in patients taking antihypertensive medications.

Complications Stroke, TIA, renal failure, CHF, acute pulmonary edema, and death.

Atlas Links UCV2 **ER-005** UCV1 PG-P1-018, PM-P1-018

5 MALIGNANT HYPERTENSION

ID/CC A 62-year-old male presents via ambulance after his wife found him lying on the floor.

HPI He is a heavy smoker who drinks excessively, is obese, and rarely exercises. His wife notes that he complained of **chest pain** and **shortness of breath** shortly before collapsing. The ambulance arrived 10 minutes after the initial event.

PE VS: no pulse; undetectable blood pressure. PE: pale; unresponsive.

Labs ECG: **[A]** ventricular fibrillation—rapid, chaotic, grossly irregular electrical activity; **[B]** sustained ventricular tachycardia—rapid (140 to 180 BPM) ventricular rate with dissociated atrial activity.

Pathogenesis Most cardiac arrests that occur by ventricular fibrillation (VF) begin with ventricular tachycardia (VT) that degenerates into fibrillation. VF is the most common electrical dysfunction and has a **short duration** before death ensues. Such disturbances can commonly occur within 24 hours of MI. The onset of VF leading to cardiac arrest is abrupt and difficult to predict.

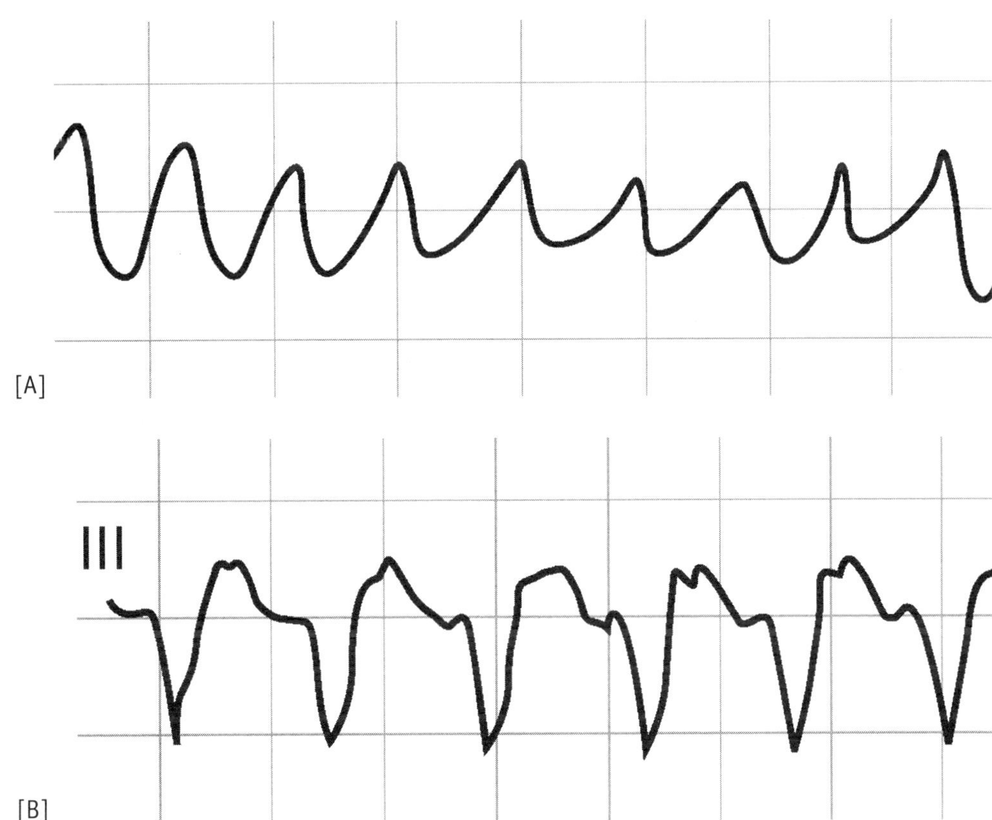

Continuous ECG monitoring in such patients may demonstrate relevant changes.

Epidemiology VF is the most common electrical mechanism underlying cardiac arrest (accounting for 75% of all such events).

Management **Immediate defibrillation** is the only intervention that can save a patient in VF. The **success of the resuscitative effort** is related to the **time elapsed from the onset of cardiac arrest**. Success rates for resuscitation depend on the age and underlying health status of the patient. Lack of CPR within the first 4 to 6 minutes of VF onset is associated with a poor outcome. Survival is good for patients who suffer a primary VF in response to acute ischemia. Survival is significantly diminished when VF is secondary to CHF, shock, MI, ventricular aneurysm, or bundle branch block. Pharmacology may include amiodarone, lidocaine, magnesium, or bretylium.

Complications Death.

MINICASE 4: CLONIDINE TOXICITY

An α_2-agonist that decreases centrally mediated sympathetic outflow and is commonly used for the treatment of hypertension, atrial fibrillation, opiate and alcohol withdrawal, nicotine addiction, migraine headaches, and Tourette's syndrome

- at therapeutic doses, side effects include dry mouth, dizziness, sedation, and constipation
- toxicity appears soon after ingestion and presents with CNS and respiratory depression, seizures, hyporeflexia, cardiac arrhythmias, hypotension, and bradycardia
- clonidine levels do not correlate with toxicity
- treat toxicity with orogastric lavage (for patients presenting within 1 hour of ingestion), charcoal (if patients present within 4 hours of ingestion), and supportive care (maintaining airway, breathing, and circulation as well as pressor support and mechanical ventilation as needed)
- prognosis is good with early presentation and prompt treatment

CARDIOLOGY

MINICASE 5: DEFIBRILLATION—AUTOMATIC EXTERNAL (AED)

Patients must be pulseless or medically unstable before an AED is applied

- electrodes are placed at the cardiac apex and the right sternal border while cardiac rhythm is monitored every 2 to 4 seconds (if the QRS complex is determined to be abnormal, then the machine delivers a biphasic shock of 115 J)
- several studies have shown that when compared to basic CPR alone, AEDs increase the survival rates of patients in ventricular fibrillation
- complications include shocking of medical personnel and local burns on the skin of the patient

MINICASE 6: DEFIBRILLATION—AUTOMATIC INTERNAL (AICD)

An implantable device that senses tachydysrhythmias (as determined by a preprogrammed acceptable rate) and responds by delivering a shock of a preset voltage

- ICDs may also attempt a series of 10 pulses in an attempt to pace-terminate the ventricular tachycardia
- newer devices are combined ICDs and pacemakers in one unit, wherein several modes are available that allow for various combinations of pacing and defibrillation of the atria and ventricles
- complications include operative failures from weak batteries or damaged wires, sensing/pacing failures, and inappropriate/ineffective cardioversion or defibrillation

MINICASE 7: ELECTROMECHANICAL DISSOCIATION

Formerly known as pulseless electrical activity, it refers to inadequate blood pressure despite adequate cardiac electrical activity

- due to cardiac tamponade, hypovolemia, acidosis, pulmonary embolism, etc.
- presents with catastrophic hypotension and systemic hypoperfusion
- ECG shows definitive electrical rhythm
- treat with cardiopulmonary resuscitation and correction of underlying condition
- complications include degeneration into asystole and diffuse organ infarction

MINICASE 8: HEART BLOCK

Conduction delays in the AV node and/or the His-Purkinje system that may be caused by congenital or acquired intrinsic nodal disease, increased vagal tone, myocardial infarction, myocarditis, electrolyte disturbances, or drugs

- first-degree block is often an incidental finding on ECG, with a prolonged PR interval (> 020 second)
- second-degree AV block is seen on ECG either as an increase in the PR interval with each successive beat until a beat is dropped (Mobitz type 1, Wenckebach phenomenon) or as a fixed ratio of initiated to conducted beats (Mobitz type 2)
- third-degree AV block (that which often presents with hypotension, altered mental status, and CHF) is seen on ECG as total AV dissociation with variable PR intervals, but with fixed PP and RR intervals
- laboratory studies may reveal electrolyte abnormalities, toxic drug levels, or elevated cardiac enzymes
- no treatment is needed for first-degree block, but administer atropine or temporary pacing for symptomatic second-degree block, and place patients with third-degree block in a monitored setting and evaluate for permanent pacing
- complications include atropine-induced arrhythmias, cardiovascular collapse, and death

MINICASE 9: HEAT STROKE

Life-threatening failure of thermoregulation seen in very young or very old patients and in people with chronic illnesses exposed to prolonged heat

- presents with confusion, delirium, loss of consciousness, anhidrosis, hypotension, and peripheral vasodilation
- core temperature is usually > 41°C
- elevated CK, myoglobinuria, hemoconcentration, and electrolyte abnormalities
- treat with cooling measures, IV fluids to prevent acute renal failure from rhabdomyolysis

MINICASE 10: MULTISYSTEM ORGAN FAILURE (MSOF)

Systemic organ dysfunction commonly due to sepsis, metastatic malignancy, extensive burns, trauma, or pancreatitis

- presents with any mix of altered mental status, CHF, DIC, oliguria, myonecrosis, and refractory hypoxia
- elevated creatinine, hyperbilirubinemia, elevated D-dimer, prolonged PT, widened A-a gradient, and elevated CK
- CXR shows diffuse pulmonary edema
- treat with emergent intubation with high O_2 and PEEP ventilatory support, vigorous fluid and pressor support to maintain hemodynamic stability, treatment of underlying condition, diuresis to maintain urine output
- poor prognosis

MINICASE 11: PROSTHETIC VALVE ENDOCARDITIS

Infection of the heart valves after surgery

- when presenting within 2 months of surgery, it is commonly caused by *Staphylococcus epidermidis* or fungal contamination of wound site
- later presentations are caused by viridans group streptococci, *S. epidermidis*, or fastidious gram-negative rods
- presents with subacute onset of fever, night sweats with diffuse embolic disease, and heart murmur
- elevated ESR
- echo reveals valvular vegetation
- treat with surgical replacement of valve and 4 to 6 weeks of a penicillin or cephalosporin, rifampin with or without aminoglycoside
- complications include valve dehiscence

MINICASE 12: SHOCK—HYPOVOLEMIC

Impaired vital organ perfusion due to a reduction in circulating blood volume (from hemorrhage or fluid depletion due to dehydration, burns, or GI fluid loss)

- presents with hypotension (MAP < 60 mmHg), tachycardia, oliguria, impaired mental status, and cool, mottled extremities
- ABGs reveal contraction alkalosis and later metabolic acidosis
- treat in the ICU with fluid replacement, packed RBCs
- prognosis is dependent on etiology and severity

MINICASE 13: SUPERIOR VENA CAVA SYNDROME

Gradual extrinsic compression of the superior vena cava, resulting in increased venous pressure, facial edema, and dilated veins

- usually caused by malignancy, commonly bronchogenic cancer or lymphoma
- presents with facial engorgement, nonpulsatile jugular venous distention, and dilated veins over the neck and chest that fill from above downward
- may need radiotherapy and treatment of the underlying cause
- complications include cardiorespiratory failure and death

MINICASE 14: THORACIC AORTIC ANEURYSM

Localized dilatation of the thoracic aorta, most often due to atherosclerosis

- asymptomatic or presents with chest pain and a history of hypertension
- CXR shows mediastinal widening
- CT and US reveal dilated aorta
- treat with surgical excision of the aneurysm with graft replacement if symptomatic, $>$ 6 cm diameter, or rapid increase in size; otherwise monitor with close follow-up

MINICASE 15: TIETZE'S SYNDROME

Costochondritis

- presents with chest pain that worsens with inspiration
- may be able to elicit pain by local palpation
- treat symptomatically with NSAIDs

MINICASE 16: VENTRICULAR FLUTTER

Ventricular arrhythmia with a rate of 150 to 300 BPM associated with ischemia or hypoxia, closely related to ventricular fibrillation

- presents with acute hypotension and hemodynamic compromise or sudden death (75% of cases of sudden death are attributed to ventricular tachycardia or to ventricular fibrillation)
- ECG shows a regular, sinusoidal undulation without distinct P-QRS-T morphology
- management is immediate defibrillation with fluid and pressor infusion to support perfusion

ID/CC A 48-year-old female presents with **sudden-onset high fever** and **generalized blistering and desquamation of the skin**.

HPI The patient has been taking **sulfonamides** for a UTI. She has no other relevant medical history and no history of allergies.

PE VS: **high fever** (39.8°C); tachycardia. PE: **ill-appearing**; areas of **ulceration in conjunctiva, nasal mucosa, mouth, oropharynx, and vagina**; eyelids swollen and erythematous; **generalized symmetric rash** on skin, primarily on **extensor surfaces**; rash accompanied by diffuse areas of denudation (epidermis completely separated from dermis).

Labs CBC: mild leukocytosis with lymphocytosis. Elevated ESR. UA: proteinuria; hematuria; numerous WBCs (due to UTI).

Imaging CXR: normal.

Pathogenesis Stevens–Johnson syndrome (a form of erythema multiforme) is an acute, severe, and **life-threatening hypersensitivity reaction** that is mediated by immune complexes. It is characterized by generalized skin **desquamation** and severe **ulcers and bullae on at least two mucosal surfaces**, including the mouth, conjunctiva, nose, and lips. **Infections** (EBV, mycoplasmal pneumonia, herpes simplex) and **drugs** (sulfa, penicillin, NSAIDs, carbamazepine, penicillamine, barbiturates, phenytoin) are the two most common causes.

Epidemiology Connective tissue disorders are associated with a higher incidence of Stevens–Johnson syndrome.

Management **Admit** to the hospital. **Discontinue the offending agent** (sulfonamides) and give **topical viscous lidocaine and IV steroids** (although use is controversial); apply Burow's solution and silver sulfadiazine cream. Porcine xenografts may be useful.

Complications Infection occurs commonly. Occasionally patients develop full-body epidermal involvement (TOXIC EPIDERMAL NECROLYSIS). Can be fatal.

STEVENS–JOHNSON SYNDROME

MINICASE 17: BULLOUS PEMPHIGOID

A pruritic skin disease usually seen in elderly patients
- presents with tense bullae that rarely rupture
- IgG and C3 at the dermal-epidermal junction on direct immunofluorescence
- treat with corticosteroids

Atlas Link: UCV2 MC-017

MINICASE 18: ERYTHEMA MULTIFORME

A self-limiting rash caused by a drug reaction (often to sulfonamides, penicillin, or phenytoin) or to certain infections (herpes simplex, *Mycoplasma pneumoniae*)
- the rash consists of erythematous target-shaped lesions that are typically worse on the trunk
- treatment involves cessation of drug intake or acyclovir to abort herpes outbreak, corticosteroids
- complications include Stevens–Johnson syndrome

Atlas Link: UCV2 MC-018

MINICASE 19: PEMPHIGUS

An intraepidermal blistering disease of the skin and mucous membranes, usually in young to middle-aged adults
- presents with painful, flaccid bullae that rupture easily, leaving denuded skin
- lesions show lateral extension and epidermal separation with rubbing
- antibody stains within epidermis on immunofluorescence
- treat with corticosteroids, add cyclophosphamide for severe disease

Atlas Links: UCV2 MC-019 UCV1 PM-P1-043

MINICASE 20: TOXIC EPIDERMAL NECROLYSIS

A severe form of skin necrosis frequently involving most of the skin surface, caused by drugs and graft-versus-host disease, not infection
- presents with epidermal separation with skin rubbing (Nikolsky's sign)
- treat with IV fluids to prevent dehydration and sterile, moist bandaging of skin
- complications include secondary infection

MINICASE 21: URTICARIA

Intradermal edema caused by an IgE-mediated allergic reaction to food or drugs

- presents with acute-onset, well-demarcated, raised erythematous wheals with central blanching
- intensely pruritic
- treatment consists of cessation of stimulatory activity (e.g., drug intake, food intake) and antihistamines for symptomatic relief
- the condition is usually self-limiting

Atlas Link: UCV2 **MC-021**

ID/CC A 14-year-old male presents with leg pains, **nausea, vomiting, abdominal pain, fever, profound weakness**, and lightheadedness a few hours **following surgery**.

HPI He is an asthmatic who has been taking **prednisone for 3 years**. He just **underwent surgery** for acute appendicitis but did not receive preoperative steroids.

PE VS: **hypotension** (BP 90/50); **fever** (38.7°C). PE: **dehydrated, confused**, and disoriented; no cardiopulmonary abnormalities; abdomen soft with no masses or rebound tenderness; no evidence of bleeding, infection, or dehiscence of surgical wound.

Labs CBC: **anemia; neutropenia; lymphocytosis; eosinophilia**. Lytes: **hyponatremia; hyperkalemia; hypochloremia. Hypoglycemia; low cortisol levels**; increased BUN. ABGs: **metabolic acidosis**. UA: **increased urinary sodium**. **ACTH low** (it would be high in primary adrenal insufficiency).

Imaging CXR: heart small in size for age.

Pathogenesis This is a **medical emergency** that may occur in patients with chronic adrenal insufficiency (ADDISON'S DISEASE); it may also be due to sudden discontinuation of chronic steroids (due to ACTH suppression) or to increased demands due to illness, fasting, heat stroke, bleeding, surgery, or trauma. Addison's disease is most frequently caused by autoimmune mechanisms; other causes include tuberculosis, adrenal hemorrhage, sarcoidosis, amyloidosis, hemochromatosis, cancer, and AIDS. The melanocyte-stimulating hormone effects of ACTH produce hyperpigmentation of the skin and mucosae. In secondary adrenal insufficiency, hyperpigmentation is not present.

Management **IV hydrocortisone** is the mainstay of acute therapy but must later be switched to oral prednisone. Since the full effect of hydrocortisone is sometimes delayed for up to 1 hour, use **dopamine** if necessary to maintain blood pressure. Treat hypoglycemia, hyponatremia, and volume depletion with IV normal saline and glucose. Prevent acute adrenal insufficiency that may arise in stressful situations with extra doses of steroids.

Complications Fatal hypoglycemia and hypotension.

ACUTE ADRENAL CRISIS

ID/CC A 35-year-old female complains of increasing **agitation and anxiety** with **confusion, vomiting, and diarrhea**.

HPI She has a **sister with myasthenia gravis, a brother with diabetes**, and an **aunt with SLE**. She has had a 6-kg **weight loss** despite an increased appetite and has also experienced **palpitations and intolerance to heat**. She recently suffered from a **severe URI**.

PE VS: **tachycardia** (HR 120); **pulse irregularly irregular** (due to atrial fibrillation); hypertension (BP 150/95); **high fever** (40.1°C). PE: **irritable** and **diaphoretic**; skin warm and moist; **exophthalmos**; neck is supple and shows **diffuse enlargement of thyroid gland** (GOITER); decreased breath sounds on right lung base with rales (due to pneumonia); brisk DTRs.

Labs CBC: leukocytosis with neutrophilia (due to pulmonary infection). Increased serum T_4 and decreased TSH (they may be normal). ECG: **atrial fibrillation**.

Imaging CXR: right lower lobe pneumonia.

Pathogenesis Also called thyrotoxic crisis, thyroid storm is an acute emergency characterized by excessive thyroid function. It may be caused by **undertreated hyperthyroidism** or may result from a **stressful situation** in a patient with **subclinical or undiagnosed hyperthyroidism**. Any event that causes stress may induce thyroid storm in a patient with subclinical disease, so clinical suspicion for underlying MI, pulmonary embolism, UTI, or diabetic ketoacidosis must be high.

Epidemiology Thyroid storm is seen with decreasing frequency, with most cases occurring in patients with Graves' disease; it carries a **high mortality rate**.

Management **Propylthiouracil** inhibits thyroid hormone synthesis and blocks peripheral conversion of T_4 to T_3. **Iodide** inhibits the release of thyroid hormone. **Steroids** inhibit the release of hormone and block the peripheral conversion of T_4 to T_3; they are also useful because of the relative adrenal insufficiency that results from the hypermetabolic state. **Propranolol** is given for severe tachycardia but should be used with caution in the presence of asthma and CHF. **Digoxin** should be given for atrial fibrillation and CHF. **Control temperature** with ice packs or acetaminophen

9 THYROID STORM

(salicylates are contraindicated because they displace thyroid hormone from thyroid-binding globulin, increasing free hormone).

Complications CHF, fatal arrhythmias, malignant hyperpyrexia, convulsions, coma, and death.

MINICASE 22: HYPOTHYROIDISM—MYXEDEMA COMA

A complication of severe hypothyroidism, usually precipitated by infection
- common in elderly females
- presents with hypothermia, hypoventilation, hypotension, hyponatremia, hypoxia, and hypercapnia
- treat with levothyroxine; intubate if necessary

MINICASE 23: LACTIC ACIDOSIS

Elevated lactic acid in blood due to shock or sepsis
- presents with tachycardia, often hypotension, tachypnea, and altered mental status
- increased serum lactate and increased anion-gap acidosis
- treat precipitating causes, administer IV fluids and pressors as needed

MINICASE 24: METABOLIC ACIDOSIS

Decreased arterial blood pH and serum bicarbonate
- classified according to anion gap, which may be decreased (plasma cell dyscrasias or hypoalbuminemia), normal (RTA, diarrhea, or loss of bicarbonate), or increased (DKA, lactic acidosis, salicylate intoxication, ethylene glycol poisoning, methanol toxicity, uremia, INH toxicity)
- presents with compensatory hyperventilation and, when severe, Kussmaul respirations
- labs reveal low blood pH, serum bicarbonate, and Pco_2, and hyperkalemia may be present
- treatment includes correcting the underlying cause
- bicarbonate may be used to treat distal RTA or severe acidosis

MINICASE 25: METABOLIC ALKALOSIS

Elevated arterial pH with increased bicarbonate due to volume contraction, excess mineralocorticoid activity, diuretic use, or alkali administration

- presents with signs/symptoms of hypovolemia (if present) or hypokalemia
- elevated arterial pH and bicarbonate levels, increased arterial Pco_2 (respiratory compensation), hypokalemia and hypochloremia may be present
- treat volume contraction with saline administration and potassium supplementation, treat aldosterone excess with potassium supplementation and ACE inhibitor or spironolactone
- complications include cardiac dysrhythmias, hypokalemia, and hypovolemia

MINICASE 26: PSEUDOHYPERKALEMIA

Due to hemolysis of RBCs after blood is drawn (releases potassium)

- presents with falsely high potassium determinations
- hemolyzed specimen has serum that looks pink
- prevent by avoiding small-bore needles
- check potassium levels immediately after blood is drawn

MINICASE 27: RESPIRATORY ACIDOSIS

Results from an increased Pco_2 secondary to hypoventilation (secondary to CNS suppression, neuromuscular disorders, airway obstruction, lung disease, or ventilator dysfunction) accompanied by acute or chronic compensation with intracellular buffers

- labs reveal decreased arterial blood pH, elevated serum bicarbonate and Pco_2
- treat the underlying cause; intubate if necessary

MINICASE 28: RESPIRATORY ALKALOSIS

Results from a decreased Pco_2 secondary to hyperventilation (secondary to central stimulation, as in stroke, infection, tumor, trauma or drugs, hypoxemia, psychogenic hyperventilation, airway irritation, sepsis, cirrhosis, or incorrect ventilator setting)

- presents with lightheadness, cramps, perioral numbness, and altered mental status
- ABGs reveals increased arterial blood pH with reduced Pco_2 and serum bicarbonate
- treat the underlying cause

ID/CC A **65-year-old** woman complains of **acute onset** of severe right **eye pain** and **frontal headache** that began while she was sitting in a movie theater.

HPI She has **blurred vision**, sees **halos around lights**, and feels very **nauseated**. She had no recent eye trauma and does not wear contact lenses. She was previously feeling well and had no antecedent headache or fever. She denies any motor weakness or vertigo and has no history of collagen vascular or inflammatory bowel disease.

PE VS: normal. PE: in mild discomfort; had an episode of **emesis** in exam room; right eye 20/100, left eye 20/40 **(decreased visual acuity)**; right eye has **conjunctival injection; pupil fixed in mid-dilation; hazy cornea**; slit-lamp exam reveals no foreign body; **shallow anterior chamber** without cells or flare; **elevated intraocular pressure** in right eye.

Pathogenesis Acute angle-closure glaucoma occurs in anatomically predisposed eyes with shallow anterior chambers. Acute **increased intraocular pressure** occurs when the **pupil is dilated** as the iris pushes against the trabecular meshwork and obstructs outflow. This is usually precipitated by topical **mydriatics, anticholinergic drugs** (e.g., antihistamines, antidepressants), **dark environments**, or **stress**.

Epidemiology Acute angle-closure glaucoma is more common in patients with farsightedness (HYPEROPIA). The elderly are predisposed owing to physiologic enlargement of the lens. Adhesions (SYNECHIAE) from previous ocular inflammation are another predisposing factor.

Management **Topical beta-blockers** (timolol, which decreases production of aqueous humor) and **topical miotics** (pilocarpine, which constricts the pupils) are used. IV **acetazolamide** (carbonic anhydrase inhibitor to decrease aqueous humor production) and **mannitol** (decreases intraocular pressure via osmotic diuresis) are also used. For definitive treatment, surgical or laser peripheral iridotomy may be performed.

Complications Permanent visual loss.

ACUTE ANGLE-CLOSURE GLAUCOMA

ID/CC A 47-year-old male presents with **pain and discharge from the right ear** and **localized pruritus**.

HPI The patient denies any fever or chills. He recently returned from a weekend of **swimming** at the beach. The pain worsens with chewing (movement of the pinna), and he notes mild decreased hearing in the affected ear. He denies having a sore throat or URI symptoms and has experienced no vertigo, nausea/vomiting, or tinnitus.

PE VS: normal. PE: tender auricle with no erythema or swelling; no mastoid tenderness; erythema and swelling of external auditory canal with whitish-yellow exudate; tympanic membrane with no erythema; oropharynx clear with no erythema, exudates, or masses; no cervical lymphadenopathy.

Labs No labs are necessary unless the patient is diabetic, in which case a CBC and glucose are warranted.

Imaging No imaging is necessary unless mastoiditis is suspected.

Pathogenesis Also called **"swimmer's ear,"** otitis externa is an **infection of the skin of the external auditory canal** that does not involve middle ear structures. It is usually caused by ***Staphylococcus aureus, Pseudomonas aeruginosa***, or *Proteus*; fungal infection with *Aspergillus* or *Candida* is also common.

Epidemiology There is a higher frequency of external otitis cases in summer, when **swimming** is more common. Overly zealous cleaning of the ear causes direct irritation and loss of protective cerumen. **Local trauma** and the irritating effects of chronic otitis media may damage the sensitive external auditory canal. **Psoriasis and seborrheic dermatitis** predispose to external ear infections.

Management Treat with **local steroid and antibiotic drops** (polymyxin, bacitracin, neomycin), analgesics, and thorough cleaning and debridement. **Systemic antibiotics** should be administered as empiric therapy for otitis media if examination of the tympanic membrane is not possible owing to exudate or significant swelling (a cotton wick may be introduced in such cases). Avoid water for 2 to 3 weeks.

Complications Malignant otitis externa (commonly seen in diabetics and usually due to *Pseudomonas aeruginosa*) may lead to facial nerve **palsy, osteomyelitis**, intracerebral abscess, septic cerebral thromboembolism, meningitis, and sepsis.

11 OTITIS EXTERNA

ID/CC A 3-year-old boy presents with a 2-day history of **fever** and **pulling on his right ear**.

HPI He is an otherwise-healthy child who is up to date with his immunizations. He suffered from a **URI 2 weeks ago**.

PE VS: **fever** (38.4°C). PE: alert but restless; pneumatic otoscopy reveals **erythema** and a **bulging tympanic membrane** with **decreased mobility** (indicating presence of fluid in the middle ear); no perforation present; oropharynx clear without exudates or erythema; no cervical lymphadenopathy.

Labs No labs are necessary unless the child appears toxic, in which case a CBC and blood culture may be warranted.

Pathogenesis Acute inflammation of the middle ear. The most common bacterial pathogens are ***Streptococcus pneumoniae***, nontypable ***Haemophilus influenzae***, and ***Moraxella catarrhalis***. Neonatal otitis media is often caused by group B streptococcus and gram-negative enterobacteria, while infants in the first 3 months of life may also become infected with *Staphylococcus aureus* and *Chlamydia trachomatis*. RSV is a common viral cause. In infants, **irritability**, constant **crying, lethargy**, and **feeding difficulties** are common presenting symptoms.

Epidemiology Acute otitis media is the **second most common infection** seen in children after the common cold. It usually follows a URI but may also appear without antecedent infection. **Breast feeding** reduces the incidence and severity of infections. **Passive smoking**, recurrent viral infections, attendance at day care centers, and later birth order predispose to infection.

Management **Amoxicillin, TMP-SMX**, or erythromycin-sulfisoxazole for 10 days; amoxicillin/clavulanate, azithromycin, and cephalosporins are reserved for refractory cases. Administer acetaminophen or ibuprofen for analgesia; topical anesthetics may also be used as long as there is no tympanic membrane perforation. Salicylates are contraindicated, since they may precipitate Reye's syndrome. Tympanocentesis and myringotomy may be needed for unresponsive cases.

Complications **Tympanic membrane perforation** and **hearing loss**, cholesteatoma formation, **mastoiditis**, cerebral abscess, meningitis, labyrinthitis, and cranial nerve palsies.

MINICASE 29: ACUTE SINUSITIS

Infection of the paranasal sinuses (most commonly the maxillary sinus) due to viral, allergic, or bacterial causes (commonly *Streptococcus pneumoniae*, *Haemophilus influenzae*, *Staphylococcus aureus*, and *Moraxella catarrhalis*)

- presents with pain in the face and upper teeth, nasal congestion and discharge, boggy nasal mucosa, and clouding of the sinuses by transillumination
- CT shows opacification of the sinuses and air-fluid levels
- treat with oral and nasal decongestants, antibiotics such as amoxicillin for bacterial sinusitis
- complications include osteomyelitis and mucocele

MINICASE 30: BENIGN POSITIONAL VERTIGO

A common form of vertigo resulting from a dislodged fragment of otolith in the semicircular canals

- presents with transient episodic vertigo associated with changes in position
- treat with repositioning exercises and antivertigo drugs

MINICASE 31: HERPES ZOSTER OPHTHALMICUS

Caused by reactivation of latent varicella virus infection in the trigeminal ganglion, with the eye invariably involved if there is evidence of nasociliary involvement (medial eyelid, conjunctiva, or tip of nose)

- presents with unilateral swelling and a vesicular rash in the skin surrounding the eye in patients with a history of childhood chickenpox
- slit-lamp examination shows coarse epithelial punctate keratitis, cornea is insensitive, vesicles have herpesvirus inclusions that are intranuclear and acidophilic (COWDRY TYPE A INCLUSION BODIES)
- treat with acyclovir and an ophthalmology consult

MINICASE 32: LABYRINTHITIS

May result from viral or bacterial infections

- typically self-limiting
- presents with abrupt onset of severe continuous vertigo, tinnitus, and hearing loss
- treat with bed rest, vestibular suppressants, and avoidance of rapid head movements

MINICASE 33: LARYNGOTRACHEOBRONCHITIS

Viral (commonly RSV) or bacterial (Mycoplasma) infection

- presents with cough, inspiratory stridor, and respiratory distress
- treat with erythromycin, bronchodilators, oxygen as needed

MINICASE 34: MASTOIDITIS

Suppurative infection of mastoid air cells (a complication of untreated otitis media)

- common causes include *Streptococcus pneumoniae*, *Haemophilus influenzae*, and *Streptococcus pyogenes*
- presents with pain in the area of the mastoid and fever
- treat with antibiotics and aggressive surgical debridement
- can progress to meningitis

MINICASE 35: OPTIC NEURITIS

Inflammation of the optic nerve, usually unilateral

- associated with demyelinating diseases such as multiple sclerosis or viral etiologies
- presents with orbital pain exacerbated by eye movement, unilateral vision loss, afferent pupillary defect, and scotomas
- treat with corticosteroids

MINICASE 36: PERITONSILLAR ABSCESS

Abscess formation in the tonsillar capsule and surrounding areas

- presents with sore throat, odynophagia, "hot potato" voice, and lockjaw
- treat with incision and drainage and antibiotics

MINICASE 37: UVEITIS

Inflammation of the iris, ciliary body, and choroid due to infection or systemic inflammation (e.g., inflammatory bowel disease)

- presents with acute, painful red eye, no loss of vision, miotic pupil, and circum-corneal ciliary congestion
- slit-lamp exam shows cells and flare in the anterior chamber
- treat with steroids, cycloplegics, and antibiotics if an infectious etiology is suspected

MINICASE 38: CHALAZION

Obstruction and sterile inflammation of the meibomian gland

- associated with seborrhea, acne rosacea, chronic blepharitis, and hyperlipidemia
- presents as a slow-growing, painless nodule on the eyelid
- most will resolve using serial warm compresses for 2 weeks
- unresolved chalazia require steroid injections by an ophthalmologist
- complications include cosmetic deformities, infection, and lid fistula

MINICASE 39: CORNEAL ABRASION

Denuding of the corneal surface caused by application of external force

- presents with severe pain, tearing, foreign body sensation, and photophobia following a history of trauma
- slit-lamp exam with fluorescein staining shows enhancement where the cornea is abraded
- ocular CT may show retained foreign body
- treat with topical anesthetics, cycloplegics, tetanus immunization, and eye rest, with most abrasions re-epithelializing within 2 days
- complications include recurrent erosions, infection, precipitation of acute narrow-angle glaucoma, and decreased visual acuity

MINICASE 40: FOREIGN BODY—EAR

Foreign bodies in the ear are usually inanimate objects or insects

- present with pain and bleeding from the ear, with swelling and a malodorous discharge indicating secondary infection
- diagnose with otoscopy
- treat with removal of the foreign body (prior to the removal of live insects, kill with mineral oil or 2% lidocaine and remove objects with irrigation, suction, or forceps using sedation if needed) and irrigation with antibiotic/steroid drops
- failure to treat promptly may lead to chronic infections and hearing loss

MINICASE 41: FOREIGN BODY—TRACHEA

Foreign bodies in the trachea (most commonly nuts, seeds, and pieces of vegetables in children and meat, bones, dental and medical appliances, and broken teeth in adults)

- usually lodge in the right main-stem bronchus and lower lobe
- present with choking, paroxysmal coughing, stridor, wheezing, and tachypnea
- adults may also show pulmonary edema
- CXR shows foreign body, atelectasis, air trapping, and mediastinal shift
- attempt removal with Heimlich maneuver, chest compressions, or back blows, maintain airway and administer oxygen while extracting by bronchoscopy
- administer steroids and antibiotics to reduce edema and infection
- complications include hypoxia, pneumonia, and abscesses

MINICASE 42: RETINAL DETACHMENT

Separation of the sensory layer of the retina from the underlying vascular choroids, most commonly caused by a break in the retina or traction on the retinal surface or by an exudate within the subretinal space

- initially presents with a sensation of flashing light (PHOTOPSIA) and floaters, progressing to a shadow in the peripheral visual field
- ophthalmoscopy shows a gray, elevated retina
- slit-lamp exam may show vitreous pigment
- US may reveal the detachment
- treat with repair using lasers, cryotherapy, or surgery
- complications include decreased visual acuity or monocular blindness

MINICASE 43: HORDEOLUM (STYE)

Localized infection (commonly with *Staphylococcus aureus*) or inflammation of an eyelash hair follicle due to obstruction of the sebaceous or meibomian glands

- associated with diabetes, blepharitis, seborrhea, and hyperlipidemia
- presents with pain, erythema, and swelling of the eyelid
- most spontaneously drain or resolve with warm compresses after 3 days, but unresolved styes require surgical drainage
- complications include orbital cellulitis, cosmetic deformities, and progression to chalazion

MINICASE 44: VITREOUS HEMORRHAGE

Bleeding into the vitreous humor caused by trauma, retinal neovascularization, or SAH

- presentation ranges from multiple floaters to dramatic loss of vision
- ophthalmoscopy may show absent red reflex with clear lens
- slit-lamp exam through dilated pupil confirms the diagnosis
- US may be needed when the view of the fundus is obstructed
- treatment involves laser cryotherapy or surgery
- prognosis depends on the underlying cause

ID/CC A **50-year-old female** presents with **severe abdominal pain and fever**.

HPI The patient has previously been diagnosed with **gallstones** and states that she has been experiencing increasing **right upper quadrant (RUQ) pain, high fevers, and jaundice** (CHARCOT'S TRIAD; if **shock and altered mental status are also present then this is termed REYNOLD'S PENTAD**). She also reports having **dark urine and clay-colored stools** (ACHOLIC STOOL).

PE VS: **fever** (39.2°C); **tachycardia** (HR 110); tachypnea (RR 26); hypotension (BP 90/60). PE: **lethargic; jaundice; icteric sclera; tender RUQ**.

Labs CBC: **leukocytosis** with left shift. LFTs: **elevated serum bilirubin and alkaline phosphatase**; transaminases elevated.

Imaging **[A]** US: **dilated common bile duct** (CBD) with obstructing stone (1). **[B]** CT, abdomen: a different case that shows **intrahepatic ductal dilatation**. Cholangiography and ERCP are relatively contraindicated during acute cholangitis. **[C]** Cholangiogram: dilated biliary tree with multiple large bile duct calculi.

Pathogenesis Ascending cholangitis is a **life-threatening emergency** resulting from **complete biliary obstruction** in the presence of **bacterial infection**. The most common causes of obstruction are **common bile duct stone** (CHOLEDOCHOLITHIASIS), **biliary stricture, and neoplasm**. The predominant bacteria in bile are *Escherichia coli, Klebsiella, Pseudomonas*, and enterococci. *Bacteroides* and other anaerobes are also present. With obstruction, the intraductal pressure increases and the bacteria proliferate, and eventually the bacteria translocate into the systemic circulation through the hepatic sinusoids. The patient exhibits clinical manifestations of sepsis.

Epidemiology The **mortality rate** for untreated or inadequately treated ascending cholangitis is 100%. Ascending cholangitis is a complication of acute choledocholithiasis. **Risk factors** are the same as for cholelithiasis (gallstones): **female gender, obesity, multiparity, age > 40 years, familial tendency**, and **chronic hemolysis**.

Management Ascending cholangitis **is a surgical emergency**. Initial therapy should consist of **IV fluids and antibiotics** (a second- or third-generation cephalosporin is the drug of choice for most

ASCENDING CHOLANGITIS

cases; if disease is severe or progressively worsens, gentamicin and clindamycin or metronidazole should be added). **Nasogastric suctioning** if persistent vomiting is present. Since choledocholithiasis is responsible for most severe cases of ascending cholangitis, **emergent endoscopic sphincterotomy** should be considered. **Prompt surgical consultation** should be obtained for operative decompression.

Complications **Hypotension**, sepsis, hepatic abscess, ARDS, and multisystem organ failure.

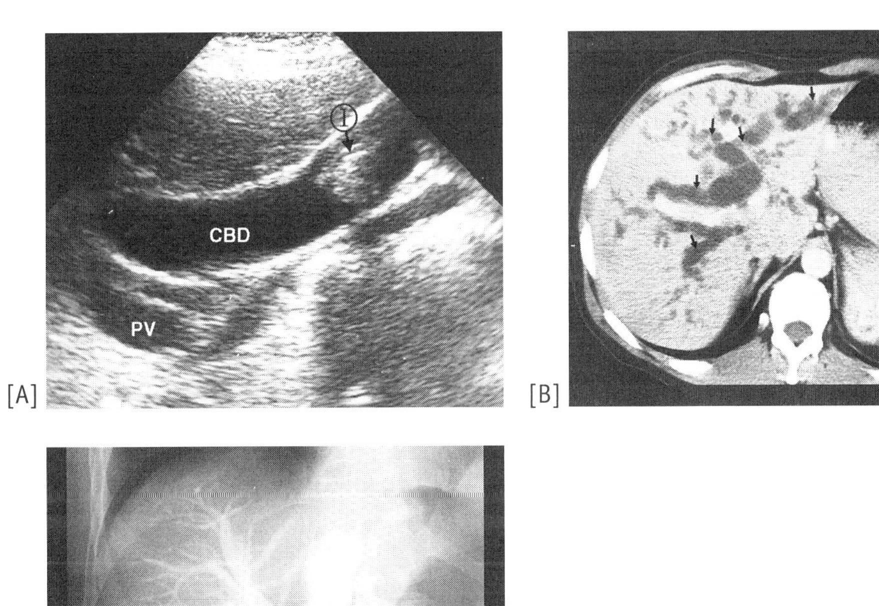

GASTROENTEROLOGY

ID/CC A **7-year-old** male presents after several episodes of **vomiting** followed by **confusion** and **tonic-clonic convulsions**.

HPI The child had been complaining of URI symptoms for the past 5 days. He was given **aspirin** for these symptoms.

PE VS: fever (39°C); tachycardia (HR 140); **tachypnea** (RR 40). PE: **delirious** and stuporous; **no jaundice**; mild bilateral **papilledema** (increased ICP); **hepatomegaly**; increased DTRs (HYPERREFLEXIA) and **Babinski's present**.

Labs CBC: **leukocytosis** with neutrophilia. **Increased serum ammonia and lactate; hypoglycemia** (with normal C-peptide levels). LFTs: markedly **elevated AST, ALT**, and **LDH**. Elevated **PT**; increased serum fatty acids. **LP: increased opening pressure**. Liver biopsy is diagnostic and shows microvesicular **fatty infiltration** with **scant inflammation**.

Imaging CT, head: no intracranial masses; marked generalized **cerebral edema**.

Pathogenesis Reye's syndrome is an acute **hepatic encephalopathy** of unknown cause that is characterized by a reversible abnormality of mitochondrial structure with decreased mitochondrial enzymatic activity (particularly the urea cycle enzymes). Viral agents **(influenza** and **varicella)** and drugs (especially **aspirin**) have been implicated as possible etiologic agents.

Epidemiology Predominantly affects children aged 6 months to 15 years.

Management Requires ICU admission. **Discontinue aspirin**; give 10% glucose for hypoglycemia, mannitol and dexamethasone for increased ICP, and fresh frozen plasma and vitamin K for coagulation defects. Correct fluid and electrolyte imbalances; avoid overhydration (increases ICP).

Complications Pancreatitis, diabetes insipidus or SIADH, aspiration pneumonia, fluid/electrolyte imbalance, arrhythmias, GI bleeding, renal failure, and respiratory failure.

MINICASE 45: FOREIGN BODY INGESTION

Most foreign bodies pass through the GI system, but common sites of impaction are the esophagus, pylorus, and ileocecal valve

- factors predisposing to an impaction are repaired tracheoesophageal fistulas, pyloric stenosis, Meckel's diverticulum, and motility disorders
- presentation depends on the site of impaction, with esophageal signs including dysphagia, food refusal, foreign body sensation, or chest/throat pain
- impactions within the stomach or lower GI tract may present with abdominal pain, distention, vomiting, hematochezia, and fever
- physical exam may show peritonitis, hematemesis, or hematochezia
- x-rays, barium studies, or endoscopy to demonstrate presence and site of foreign body
- removal may be spontaneous or performed with endoscopy, catheterization, or surgery
- complications include abrasions, strictures, perforation, and infection

MINICASE 46: ESOPHAGEAL SPASM

May be related to acid reflux irritation but is often idiopathic

- presents with acute, retrosternal burning or crushing pain similar in quality to angina
- often occurs during ingestion of food or liquid, but may occur during exercise
- esophageal manometry demonstrates pressure oscillations secondary to spasm, UGI shows "corkscrew" esophagus
- treat with calcium channel blockers, nitroglycerin, or esophageal myotomy for refractory cases
- complications include development of achalasia

MINICASE 47: FOREIGN BODY—RECTUM

Foreign bodies in the rectum are usually inserted but may be swallowed

- they are classified as high-lying or low-lying in relation to the rectosigmoid junction
- presents with abdominal pain or rectal pain and bleeding
- rectal exam should be deferred until the location and type of foreign body have been determined
- CBC may indicate infection or hemorrhage, AXRs will help identify the object and rule out a perforation
- extraction may be attempted with forceps or surgery
- complications include perforation, infection, abscess, and sepsis

MINICASE 48: FULMINANT HEPATIC FAILURE

Defined as the development of hepatic encephalopathy within 8 weeks of onset of acute liver disease, commonly due to acute viral hepatitis (mostly HBV, HEV in endemic areas, HAV, and rarely HCV), drugs (acetaminophen, valproate, isoniazid, halothane), shock, malignancy, Reye's syndrome, and acute fatty liver of pregnancy

- presents with rapidly progressing nausea/vomiting, abdominal pain, hemorrhage, and hepatic encephalopathy
- marked elevation of transaminases, hyperbilirubinemia, prolonged PT, and metabolic abnormalities (hypoglycemia, azotemia, acid-base and electrolyte imbalances)
- treat supportively for correction of metabolic abnormalities
- treat hepatic encephalopathy (zero protein diet, avoidance of precipitating factors and drugs, lactulose, antibiotics)
- monitor and treat cerebral edema (mannitol), early administration of N-acetylcysteine to abort acetaminophen-induced necrosis
- liver transplantation is required to prevent death once necrosis occurs

MINICASE 49: GASTROENTERITIS

Most commonly due to gram-negative rods (e.g., *Campylobacter, Escherichia coli, Salmonella*), protozoa (*Giardia, Entamoeba, Cryptosporidium*), or viruses (rotavirus, echovirus)

- presents with abdominal cramping and purulent diarrhea, possibly bloody, lasting 1 to 2 weeks before resolving
- stool WBCs are elevated
- cultures may reveal organism
- parasites seen on smear
- treat with fluids as needed, fluoroquinolone can be used to shorten the course of the disease
- complications include dehydration and hemorrhage in severe enteroinvasive disease

MINICASE 50: HEMORRHAGIC GASTRITIS—DRUG-INDUCED

Caused by ingestion of corrosive substances, corticosteroids, alcohol, or aspirin, or secondary to severe systemic stress

- presents with nausea, vomiting, epigastric pain, coffee-ground emesis, tachycardia, and hypotension
- anemia and occult blood in stool
- UGI reveals erosions and fold thickening, EGD reveals petechial hemorrhages and small mucosal ulcerations
- treat with antacids, IV fluids, and transfusion as needed
- complications include hemodynamic collapse

MINICASE 51: HEPATIC ENCEPHALOPATHY

Delirium secondary to hepatic failure

- presents with asterixis and a global decline in cognition and orientation
- metabolic abnormalities (hypoglycemia, electrolyte and acid-base imbalances, azotemia), elevated transaminases and serum ammonia levels, hyperbilirubinemia, and prolonged PT
- treat with restriction of protein intake, avoidance of precipitating factors (GI bleeding, infections, hypokalemia, alkalosis, diuretics, sedatives such as benzodiazepines), correction of metabolic abnormalities, lactulose and neomycin to lower ammonia levels, monitoring and treatment of cerebral edema
- consider liver transplant
- complications include cerebral edema leading to herniation and death

MINICASE 52: SPONTANEOUS BACTERIAL PERITONITIS

A bacterial infection of ascitic fluid (commonly in the presence of cirrhosis or nephrotic syndrome)

- in the absence of an apparent intra-abdominal source, usually due to hematogenous spread
- most commonly caused by *Escherichia coli, Klebsiella pneumoniae*, enterococcus, or gram-positive bacteria
- presents with abdominal pain and low-grade fever in patients with cirrhotic ascites or nephrotic syndrome
- ascitic fluid PMN count > 250 cells/μL, ascitic fluid culture positive for bacterial organism
- abdominal USG shows ascites
- treat with third-generation cephalosporins (usually cefotaxime) and prevent recurrences with oral fluoroquinolone prophylaxis

ID/CC A **70-year-old male** is seen after having a **syncopal episode** accompanied by **acute-onset abdominal pain**.

HPI The patient is a heavy **smoker** with a history of **hypertension**. His wife states that before he passed out, he complained of abdominal pain **radiating to his back**.

PE VS: tachycardia (HR 120); tachypnea (RR 26); **hypotension** (BP 90/60). PE: diaphoretic; in severe distress; abdominal exam reveals **tender pulsatile abdominal mass** (present in 75% of patients) with an audible **abdominal bruit; decreased pulses in lower extremities**.

Labs Normal.

Imaging **[A]** XR, abdomen: curvilinear calcification in a large abdominal aortic aneurysm (AAA) (not sensitive; not performed acutely). **[B]** CT, abdomen: a different case with a nonruptured large AAA with a calcified wall (1) and an intramural thrombus (2). **[C]** US, abdomen: another AAA with thrombus.

Pathogenesis An **aneurysm is defined as a dilatation of a vessel by > 50%**. The normal abdominal aorta is approximately 2 cm in diameter; therefore, a 3-cm abdominal aorta is considered an aneurysm. AAAs are multifactorial in origin but show a **strong genetic predisposition**; local **mechanical forces** also play a role in aneurysm formation. Unlike the thoracic aorta, **the abdominal aorta is predisposed to true aneurysm formation** because of **turbulent flow** owing to its many branches. **Atherosclerosis** is the primary risk factor for AAA.

Epidemiology **Seventy-five percent of AAAs occur in patients older than 60 years**. There is a predominance in males, smokers, hypertensives, COPD patients, and patients with collagen vascular diseases (Marfan's and Ehlers-Danlos syndromes). AAAs are found in approximately **5% of the population older than 65 years**.

Management If the patient is asymptomatic and the aneurysm is **< 5 cm** in diameter, he or she may be safely **discharged with follow-up**. Patients with aneurysms **> 5 cm** should be referred directly to a surgeon. If the patient is symptomatic and hemodynamically stable in the ER, an **immediate surgical consultation** should be obtained. Start **two large-bore IVs; type and cross 10 units of packed RBCs**. Imaging studies (e.g., CT) should be selected on the basis of their immediate availability (CT versus ultrasound). Unstable patients need immediate surgery. The patient should be aggressively resuscitated until taken to the OR. The mortality rate for a ruptured AAA approaches 75%.

Complications **Risk of rupture is directly related to the diameter of the aneurysm**. Aneurysms < 4 cm rarely rupture; aneurysms 4 to 5 cm in diameter are associated with a 5% to 10% chance of rupturing within 5 years. This risk increases directly with the size of the aneurysm.

Atlas Link UCVI PG-P2-001

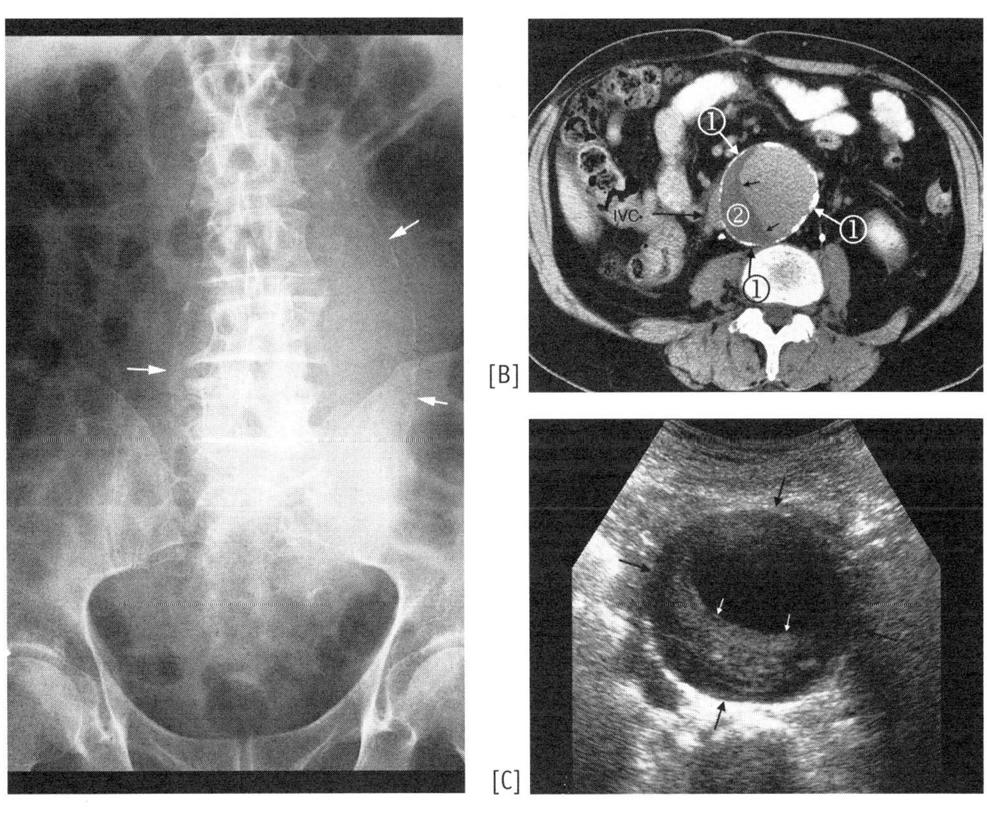

ID/CC A 2-year-old child sustained an electrical shock injury after he inserted a wire hanger into an electrical outlet.

HPI The mother states that the child could not let go of the wire and continued contact with it for a long time (due to hand muscle tetany).

PE VS: hypotension (BP 60/40); **tachycardia** (HR 120). PE: **confused**, crying, and **irritable; hand severely swollen**; thumb and index finger have **deep burns**; both knees have "outlet wound" injury (child was on his knees at time of accident).

Labs **CPK markedly elevated**. Lytes: **hyperkalemia**; hyperphosphatemia (due to muscle necrosis); hypocalcemia (due to deposition in necrotic muscle). Hyperuricemia; hypoalbuminemia; **increased creatinine; markedly increased myoglobin** in serum and urine. ECG: normal.

Imaging CXR/KUB: normal.

Pathogenesis Electric shock is usually caused by contact with **alternating current** in **the home**. High-voltage electrical wiring and lightning may also cause electric shock. The voltage, type and degree of current, resistance encountered, and duration of contact are factors that affect the outcome of the lesion. **Nerves, blood vessels, and muscles** suffer lesions from electrical current to a much higher degree than does fat or bone.

Management Treatment consists of local wound care, hydration, diuresis (with mannitol), urine alkalinization, administration of antibiotics such as penicillin (to prevent clostridial infection), and treatment of hyperkalemia and other electrolyte imbalances. Evaluate the need for **fasciotomy** (in case of neurovascular compromise). Give tetanus prophylaxis. Hemodialysis is indicated in severe cases.

Complications Complications include **ventricular fibrillation, cardiopulmonary arrest**, vertebral and rib fractures, joint dislocations, respiratory depression, loss of consciousness, and tendon avulsions. Myoglobinuria and reduced renal perfusion from volume depletion may cause **acute tubular necrosis**.

ID/CC A 2-year-old **male** is seen for **acute onset** of severe, **colicky**, intermittent **abdominal pain** and **passage of mucus mixed with blood** per rectum (CURRANT JELLY STOOL).

HPI On his way to the hospital, he **vomited** three times.

PE VS: **tachycardia** (HR 150); tachypnea (RR 44); mild **fever** (38.8°C). PE: pallor; crying; abdomen tender, **distended**, and tympanic; firm, **sausage-shaped mass** palpated in right abdomen; rectal exam discloses **blood and mucus on examining finger**; child has bouts of pain with **intermittent** periods of relief.

Labs CBC: **leukocytosis with neutrophilia**. ABGs: metabolic alkalosis (vomiting of HCl). Lytes: hypokalemia.

Imaging **[A]** KUB: film taken during air-insufflated reduction shows a filling defect in the colon from invaginated ileum. **[B]** BE: obstruction in the mid-transverse colon. During barium enema, the intussusception was relieved spontaneously with free passage of barium proximally (hydrostatic reduction).

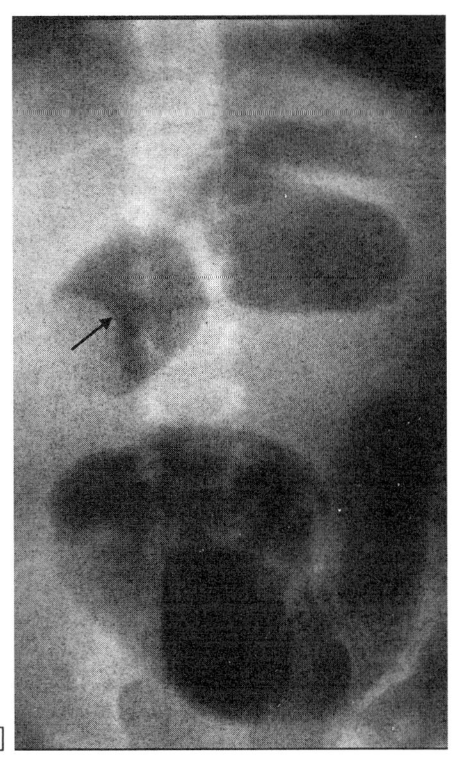

[A]

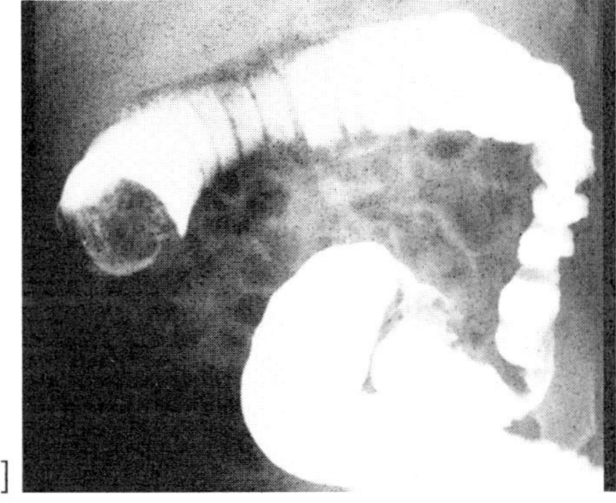

[B]

INTUSSUSCEPTION

Pathogenesis Intussusception is invagination of a portion of intestine into a distal segment. The most common type of intussusception is ileocolic. Although it is usually **idiopathic**, polyps, tumors, inflamed Peyer's patches, Meckel's diverticulum, or other masses can act as lead points. Obstruction leads to mucosal edema, sloughing, impairment of venous and then arterial supply, necrosis, gangrene, and perforation. Intussusception typically presents as **paroxysmal colicky** abdominal pain, **"currant jelly" stools**, and mass in the ileocolic region.

Epidemiology The most common cause of intestinal obstruction in young children between the ages of 3 months and 6 years. Peaks at **6 to 18 months**; has **male predominance** (male-to-female ratio is 4:1).

Management Attempt **hydrostatic reduction** via a water-soluble contrast enema (50% successful; contraindicated if peritoneal signs are present). **Surgical** treatment consists of intraoperative manual reduction. If unsuccessful, resection with primary anastomosis should be performed. Postoperative complications include anastomotic leakage and prolonged ileus.

Complications Recurrence in 5% to 10% of patients, usually within the first 48 hours after barium enema reduction.

Atlas Link UCV1 PG-P2-009

MINICASE 53: FROSTBITE

Ischemia and necrosis of tissues (commonly the hands and feet) secondary to cold exposure and resultant metabolic and microvascular damage

- the most severe damage occurs with slow, prolonged cold exposure
- usually seen in the homeless, outdoor workers, and winter outdoor enthusiasts
- presents with cold, burning, numb extremities
- findings range from erythema and edema to full-thickness injury affecting muscle and bones
- scintigraphy with technetium-99 indicates the extent of deep-tissue injury
- treat with rapid rewarming, antibiotics, surgical debridement, or amputation
- complications include infection, acidosis, cardiac arrhythmias, and gangrene

ID/CC A 19-year-old male was **stabbed in the abdomen** during a gang fight in his neighborhood.

HPI He drinks **alcohol** heavily at least twice a week and uses IV **drugs** regularly.

PE VS: **tachycardia** (HR 120); **hypotension** (BP 90/60); tachypnea (RR 28). PE: awake and protects airway well; strong femoral pulses present bilaterally; no head, neck, or chest trauma; abdomen has three stab wounds, one in the left upper quadrant and two in the periumbilical region; mild abdominal distention; **generalized abdominal tenderness with rebound tenderness**; decreased bowel sounds; back has no exit wounds or trauma; rectal exam is heme negative.

Labs CBC: **low hematocrit** (after crystalloid rehydration). UA: no hematuria; toxicology screen positive for cocaine. Increased serum ethanol level.

Imaging CXR: no hemopneumothorax (might show free subdiaphragmatic air in upright film if the hollow viscus is damaged). KUB: moderate generalized ileus; no foreign body. US: hemoperitoneum as evidenced by free fluid in Morrison's pouch (hepatorenal recess).

Pathogenesis Penetrating abdominal injuries **traverse the peritoneum**.

Epidemiology Generally, blunt abdominal trauma has a higher mortality rate than penetrating injuries. Use of alcohol or drugs places patients at higher risk for violence-related trauma.

Management Stabilize the patient (ABCs, place two large-bore IVs, type and cross, fluid resuscitation). **Immediate surgical exploration** is warranted for refractory hypotension, obvious evisceration, peritoneal signs, or a **positive peritoneal lavage** (macroscopic blood, > 100,000 RBCs/mm^3 for blunt trauma or > 20,000 for penetrating trauma, > 500 WBCs/mm^3, > 200 U/100 mL amylase, bile or feces in aspirate). **Gunshot wounds** should always be explored surgically.

Complications Exsanguinating hemorrhage, peritonitis, and sepsis.

PENETRATING ANTERIOR ABDOMINAL WOUND

ID/CC A 43-year-old male presents with **chest pain** and **dyspnea** after having been **stabbed** in a subway station.

HPI He is a tourist who refused to hand over his watch to muggers and was subsequently **stabbed in the right thorax** with a handknife.

PE VS: tachycardia (HR 110); tachypnea (RR 36); hypotension (BP 90/70). PE: single 2-cm-long stab wound to right chest in fifth intercostal space on anterior axillary line; **poor chest expansion** on inspiration with **hyperresonance; absence of breath sounds** and **decreased tactile fremitus** in right lung.

Labs CBC: mild leukocytosis. ABGs: **mild hypoxemia**. ECG: nonspecific ST-T changes.

Imaging **[A]** CXR: **hyperlucency of the right thorax; visceral pleural line visible; lung collapse** (PNEUMOTHORAX). **[B]** CXR: a different case in which air is seen in the mediastinum (PNEUMOMEDIASTINUM). **[C]** XR, lateral neck: a different case in which the esophagus has been perforated, leading to soft-tissue emphysema (1).

Pathogenesis Penetrating wounds of the thorax are those in which the **parietal pleura is severed**; they may give rise to the accumulation of air in the pleural space (PNEUMOTHORAX), blood in the pleural space (HEMOTHORAX), a combination of both (HEMOPNEUMOTHORAX), an accumulation of blood in the pericardial sac (HEMOPERICARDIUM), air in the mediastinum (PNEUMOMEDIASTINUM), or blood in the mediastinum (HEMOMEDIASTINUM). Lesions of the thoracic duct may give rise to chylothorax. The presence of air in the subcutaneous tissue with crepitation (SUBCUTANEOUS EMPHYSEMA) may be caused by rupture of the parietal pleura, trachea, esophagus, or bronchi. Penetrating thoracic wounds may also involve the peritoneum and may thus be "double-penetrating" lesions.

Management Foreign bodies should not be removed until possible bleeding can be controlled. Check for airway obstruction, sit the patient in Fowler's position (knees to chest) or over the affected side, and encourage coughing. Treat pain to avoid splinting. **Treat shock** with crystalloids or colloids if necessary. For flail chest, **positive intermittent pressure** with a ventilator is needed; for hemopneumothorax or pneumothorax, place a **chest tube** in the fourth intercostal space in the midaxillary line. For central chest wounds, **cardiac echo** should be used to rule out tamponade, and an **angiogram** should be ordered to evaluate the great vessels. **Surgery** is indicated for persistent hemorrhage seen on chest tube drainage.

Complications Fatal bleeding, tension pneumothorax, tamponade, aspiration, lung abscess, shock, and pneumonia.

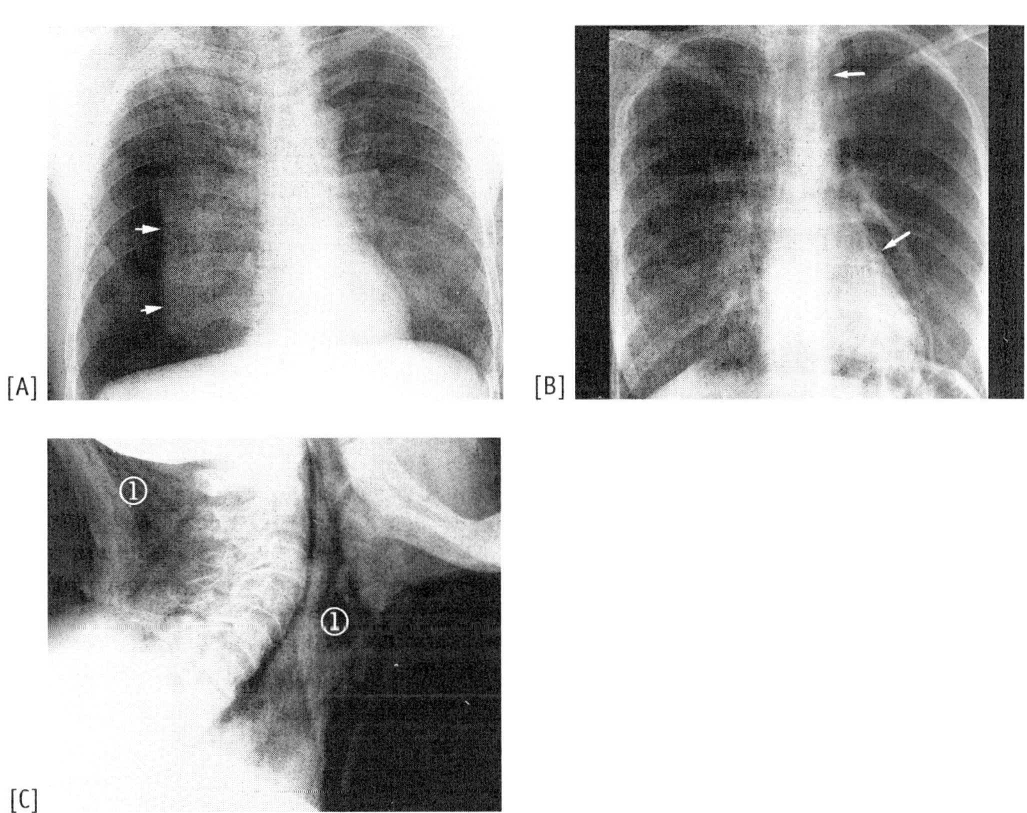

GENERAL SURGERY

ID/CC A 73-year-old **male** presents with a 5-day history of **abdominal pain, distention**, and **obstipation**.

HPI He has been suffering from **chronic constipation** for several years and **frequently uses enemas**.

PE VS: **tachycardia** (HR 110); **hypotension** (BP 90/40). PE: **dehydration; marked abdominal distention**; abdomen **tympanic; tenderness to palpation** but no muscle rigidity or rebound tenderness; generalized **mass with "air balloon" consistency felt in left abdomen** extending from pelvis to costal margin; hyperperistaltic bowel sounds; rectal vault empty.

Labs CBC: increased hematocrit (due to fluid loss); **leukocytosis** (16,550) with 76% PMNs and 10% bands. BUN and creatinine mildly elevated; amylase and lipase normal. LFTs: normal.

Imaging **[A]** KUB: typical **"inner tube" or "inverted U" image** represents great distention of the sigmoid colon from the pelvis to the diaphragm. **[B]** XR, abdomen: the typical **bird-beak** sign is seen at the level of the twisted mesentery after a Gastrografin enema. **[C]** XR, abdomen: a Gastrografin enema in another patient reveals the twisted section of sigmoid and dilatation of the colon proximal to the volvulus.

Pathogenesis Volvulus is a **rotation of the intestine** (twisting) that causes an intestinal obstruction; it **most commonly occurs in the sigmoid area** but may also occur in the small bowel and cecum. **Heredity** plays a role in its pathogenesis; a congenital defect in the length of mesentery that fixes the sigmoid colon has been proposed as a cause. **Obstruction** in volvulus is of the **closed-loop type**, i.e., there are two obstacle points for feces to transit (can't go caudad, can't go cephalad); hence, there is a **higher incidence of necrosis**.

Epidemiology **Males are affected more frequently** than females. Volvulus is second only to carcinoma as a cause of complete colonic obstruction. A **diet high in residues** of indigestible vegetable fiber increases the incidence of volvulus. **Continuous enemas**, cathartic use, infection with *Trypanosoma cruzi*, and pregnancy are associated with a higher incidence of volvulus. The clinical course is more acute in younger patients than in the elderly.

Management Pain and intestinal obstruction must be relieved with a large **rectal tube** or **rectosigmoidoscopy**. The tube must be left in place sutured to the anal margin for a few days to prevent early recurrence. Long-term recurrence is prevented through **elective resection** of the involved segment.

Complications Fluid and electrolyte imbalance, shock, gangrene, perforation, generalized peritonitis, intra-abdominal abscess formation, perforation while doing endoscopy, postoperative dehiscence of anastomosis, and recurrence.

[A]

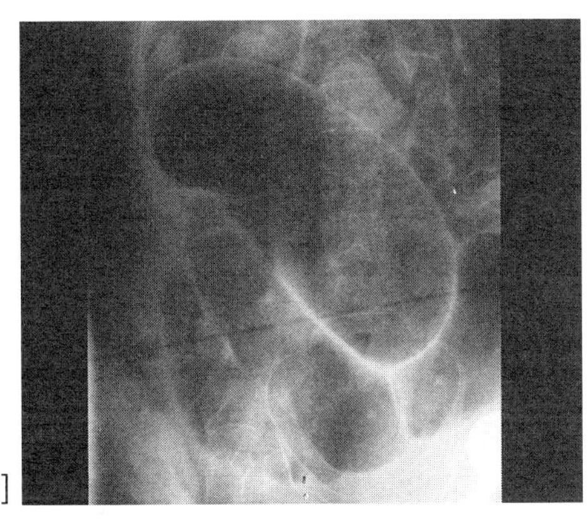

[B]

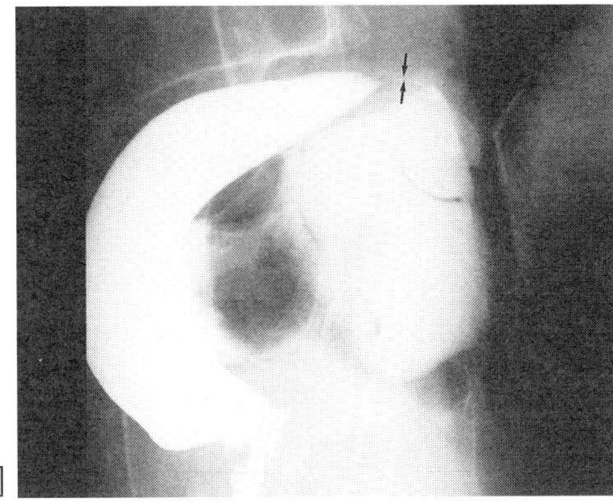

[C]

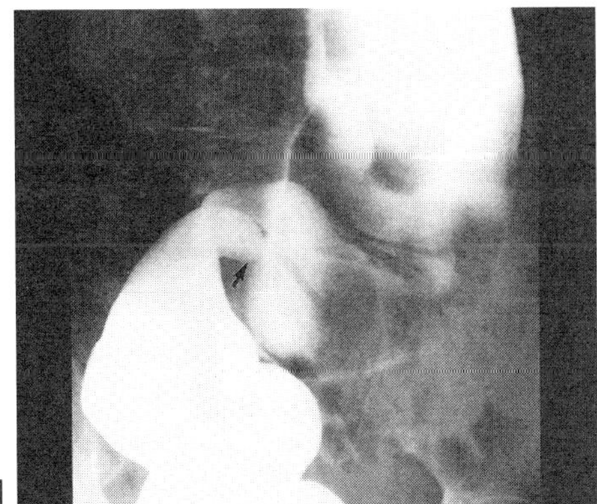

ID/CC A 25-year-old male is rescued by firefighters from a burning building; he is **coughing**, in **severe pain**, and **dyspneic**.

HPI He was found in an upstairs bedroom (**enclosed space** increases risk of inhalational injury and carbon monoxide poisoning). The **exposure time** is unknown, and there were no associated explosions (decreases suspicion for **trauma related to blast injury**). There were no **toxic materials of combustion** at the scene.

PE VS: tachycardia (HR 110); tachypnea (RR 30); normal BP; Sao_2 90% on room air. PE: moderate distress; **singed nasal hairs** with **soot in mouth** and pharynx; **carbonaceous sputum** (evidence of inhalation injury); mild perioral burns; bilateral **wheezing**; face **tender and red, resembling a sunburn** (FIRST-DEGREE BURN); chest and abdomen **red, moist, and painful with blisters throughout** (SECOND-DEGREE BURN); both lower extremities **charred, gray-appearing, and insensitive to painful stimuli** (THIRD-DEGREE BURN).

Labs ABGs: metabolic acidosis and mild **hypoxia. Carboxyhemoglobin level** elevated; serum **CK levels** elevated. UA: myoglobinuria.

Imaging CXR: to evaluate hypoxia, pneumothorax, or **pulmonary edema**. Other diagnostic imaging should be directed by suspicion of injury or trauma.

Pathogenesis Burns are defined by their **size** (% TBSA determined by the **rule of nine**) and **depth**; tissue damage is caused by **protein denaturation. First-degree burns** involve the epidermis alone. **Second-degree** burns involve the dermis (but spare some epidermal structures, such as hair follicles and sweat glands), are exquisitely painful, and are generally associated with blister formation. **Third-degree burns** are characterized by involvement of the entire skin down to the subcutaneous fat. There is extensive scarring, and the site appears charred, leathery, and **painless**, since the nerve endings have been destroyed. Third-degree burns require **surgical repair and skin grafts. Fourth-degree burns** are deep enough to involve fascia, muscle, and bone; the tissue itself is **necrotic**.

Epidemiology Burns are the **second most common cause of accidental death in the United States**. Approximately two million people present to the ER every year with thermal burn injuries; 100,000 of these are hospitalized, and about 12,000 die. The **very young**

and the elderly have the highest incidence of complications and mortality.

Management Address **ABCs** first. High-flow **oxygen** and **two large-bore IV lines** should be started immediately. **Early intubation** is indicated, since airway edema may make this impossible later. **Fluid resuscitation with lactated Ringer's** should be estimated using the **Parkland formula** (4 cc/kg per % TBSA burned/24 hrs). Half of these fluids should be given over the first 8 hours, and the second half given over the following 16 hours. A **Foley catheter** is inserted to measure urinary output. **Urinary output should be maintained at 0.5 to 1.0 cc/kg/hr. Tetanus prophylaxis** should be administered, and **IV narcotics** should be given to provide adequate pain relief. Burns should be **irrigated with saline** and covered with **sterile dressing. Topical antibiotics** (silver sulfadiazine or bacitracin) should be applied; prophylactic PO antibiotics are not indicated. Circumferential burns must be monitored closely for signs of **compartment syndrome**. Distal pulses should be monitored closely. **Escharotomy** is indicated for compromised circulation or inability to ventilate the patient.

Complications Burns are often complicated by **rhabdomyolysis, hypovolemic "burn" shock** due to intravascular volume loss resulting from poor vascular integrity, and the development of **ARDS. Infection** (especially *Pseudomonas* septicemia) is a delayed cause of death for many burn patients. Other complications include gastroduodenal erosions and ulceration **(Curling's ulcer)** due to stress.

Atlas Links UCV2 **ER-021A, ER-021B, ER-021C**

MINICASE 54: ACUTE INTERMITTENT PORPHYRIA

An autosomal-dominant deficiency of porphobilinogen deaminase, an enzyme involved in porphobilinogen metabolism

- presents with systemic symptoms, acute abdominal pain, neuropsychiatric problems, and CNS and peripheral neuropathy
- may be precipitated by sun exposure and by certain medications that induce cytochrome P-450
- UA shows increased urine porphobilinogen and γ-aminolevulinic acid
- treat with high-carbohydrate diet, glucose, hematin

ID/CC A 38-year-old female complains of **unilateral left leg swelling** that has worsened over the past 3 days.

HPI The patient states that her leg has become increasingly **painful** and **tender**. She denies having any fever, chills, or shortness of breath, and she cannot recall any trauma to the leg. She is a **smoker** and is taking **OCPs**. She works as a telephone operator and is **immobile** for long periods of time.

PE VS: low-grade fever (38.1°C). PE: **obese** and in no apparent distress; chest clear bilaterally with normal heart sounds; examination of extremities reveals a markedly swollen, warm, and tender left leg; firm elongated structure **(cord)** can be palpated in posterior calf; **pain in calf when foot is passively dorsiflexed** (HOMANS' SIGN); pulses equal.

Imaging **Duplex US** (real-time ultrasound imaging with color-flow mapping): large thrombus in the superficial femoral vein. **[A] Venogram** (considered the gold standard because of high sensitivity and specificity; disadvantage is that it is invasive): a different case in which filling defects are seen in the popliteal vein (1). **[B]** Venogram: a different case, again showing filling defects in the femoral vein (compare with the normal opacity of more proximal veins).

Pathogenesis Deep venous thromboses (DVTs) are caused by an element of **Virchow's triad** (VENOSTASIS, HYPERCOAGULABILITY, ENDOTHELIAL INJURY). The physical manifestations of DVT are determined by the extent and location of the thrombus. Massive DVT of the iliac and pelvic veins (PHLEGMASIA CERULEA DOLENS, or "painful blue inflammation") is an ischemic form of DVT in which the leg is intensely swollen and cyanotic.

Epidemiology The prevalence of DVT is directly related to the number of risk factors present. Known risk factors include **prior DVT; carcinoma**; age > 40 years; obesity; **estrogen therapy; immobility or prolonged bed rest**; recent trauma, burns, or surgery; MI; CHF; pregnancy; **and inherited abnormalities of coagulation** (most commonly activated are protein C resistance, protein S deficiency, and antithrombin III deficiency).

Management **Parenteral heparin followed by warfarin** is administered to prevent **pulmonary embolism**. PTT should be maintained between 1.5 and 2.5 times the control value. **Low-molecular-weight heparin** is equally effective in treating DVT; it requires no laboratory monitoring and can be given subcutaneously once or twice daily. **Thrombolytic therapy** may be used with heparin in patients with RV compromise or hemodynamic instability due to massive, life-threatening pulmonary embolism; tPA, urokinase, and streptokinase have all been approved for this application. Thrombolysis is associated with an **increased risk of bleeding**. Prophylaxis against DVT includes pneumatic compression for all patients undergoing surgery; subcutaneous heparin therapy for medical patients at modest risk for venous thrombosis; and warfarin or low-molecular-weight heparin for surgical patients at high risk.

Complications The primary complication of DVT is **pulmonary embolism**.

[A]

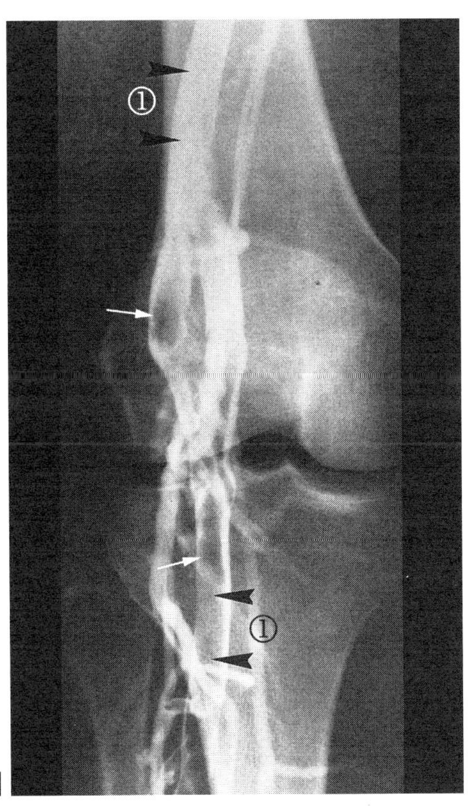

[B]

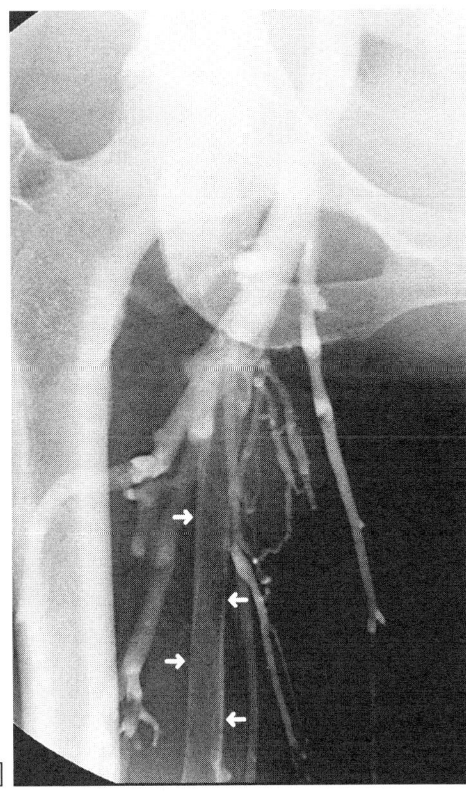

ID/CC A 13-year-old **black** female is brought to the emergency room with **acute, agonizing pain** in both legs and in the lower back.

HPI The patient has been suffering from **recurrent abdominal and joint pains** (due to ischemia) and was diagnosed as having sickle cell disease. She has required **multiple previous hospital admissions for pain and anemia management**.

PE VS: tachycardia; low-grade fever (38.1°C). PE: distress secondary to severe pain; conjunctiva pale; jaundice (due to hemolysis); funduscopic exam shows hemorrhages and **hypoxic spots with neovascularization**; mild effusion seen on both knees; spleen not palpable owing to autoinfarction.

Labs CBC: **decreased hematocrit**; mild leukocytosis. **[A]** PBS: characteristic **sickle-shaped erythrocytes**; reticulocytosis. LFTs: hyperbilirubinemia (unconjugated); increased LDH. Hemoglobin electrophoresis reveals hemoglobin F (HbF); sodium metabisulfite causes sickling of RBCs. UA: microscopic hematuria.

Imaging XR, hands and feet: soft tissue swelling with radiolucent areas (BONE NECROSIS).

Pathogenesis Sickle cell disease is an **autosomal-recessive** hemoglobinopathy (HbS) that is due to a point mutation on the gene coding for the β chain of hemoglobin. In sickle cell disease, vaso-occlusive crises occur due to sickling of RBCs, which causes occlusion of the microvasculature of different organs that in turn gives rise to painful attacks of the limbs, chest, and back and may also cause ischemic damage. Precipitating events for crises include acidosis, hypoxemia, dehydration, and infection.

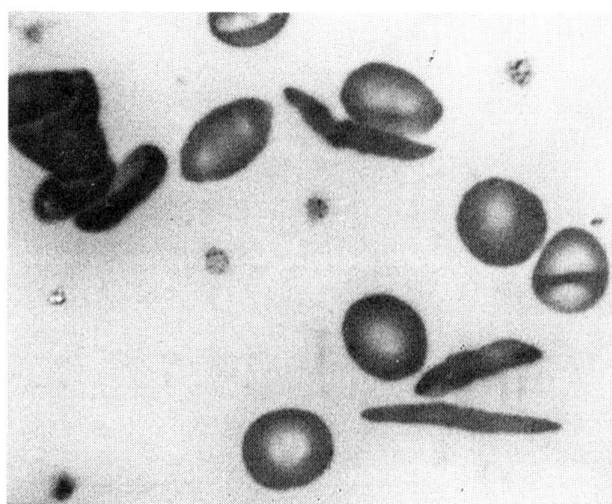
[A]

SICKLE CELL ANEMIA—VASO-OCCLUSIVE CRISIS

Epidemiology Sickle cell disease is more commonly seen in patients of African, Mediterranean, Middle Eastern, and Indian descent. It is also the **most common hemoglobinopathy in blacks**, with an incidence of 1 in 400; the trait is carried by 7% of black Americans. Homozygotes present with the disease.

Management **Vigorous IV fluid administration** due to hyposthenuria (inability to concentrate urine); give **oxygen. Control pain** with ibuprofen, morphine, or hydrocodone according to severity; avoid meperidine owing to the risk of normeperidine accumulation and seizures. Use respiratory depressants (e.g., narcotics) with caution. Transfuse if markedly anemic, administer folic acid, and treat infections with appropriate antibiotics. Hydroxyurea may increase HbF level; exchange transfusion (if $Pa_{O_2} < 60$ mmHg) and marrow transplant may be used in severe cases. Treat retinopathy with laser photocoagulation.

Complications Complications include cerebrovascular occlusive crises with hemiplegia, hepatic and pulmonary crises, priapism, renal papillary infarction, retinal detachment, cholelithiasis, septicemia due to encapsulated organisms, meningitis, pneumonia, *Salmonella* osteomyelitis, chronic leg ulcers, aseptic necrosis of the femoral head, retinal infarcts, zinc deficiency, autosplenectomy (due to repeated thrombosis), and bone infarction with necrosis. Acute crises with fever, marrow necrosis, and respiratory failure due to ischemic lung disease (ACUTE CHEST SYNDROME) may be fatal. **Parvovirus B19 infection may precipitate aplastic crises.**

MINICASE 55: HEPARIN TOXICITY

Acute hemorrhage due to overdosing or to autoimmune thrombocytopenia as a side effect of appropriate dosing

- presents with extensive ecchymoses and hemorrhage
- thrombocytopenia, markedly prolonged PTT in overdosage
- treat with discontinuation of heparin, protamine sulfate, blood and platelet transfusions as needed

ID/CC A 45-year-old female complains of **black, tarry stools** (MELENA) and **bleeding from the gums** when she brushes her teeth; she started her period yesterday and has had **profuse menstrual bleeding**.

HPI She is a diabetic with a history of aortobifemoral bypass and has been on **warfarin** for several years. **She has been taking amoxicillin for 2 days** for cellulitis of the right foot.

PE VS: **fever** (38.4°C). PE: skin and mucosa **pale; petechiae** on limbs and chest; **gums are bleeding**; good, **strong pulse in both dorsalis pedis; right foot swollen, erythematous, warm**, and **tender** to palpation.

Labs CBC: **anemia** (Hb 10.1); **leukocytosis** (15,700) with 85% neutrophils (due to cellulitis). **Elevated PT** (30); **elevated INR** (6; therapeutic level usually 2 to 3).

Imaging CXR: normal. XR, leg: increase in density of soft tissue with no bony involvement.

Pathogenesis Warfarin interferes with the synthesis of **vitamin K-dependent coagulation factors** (II, VII, IX, X). It takes up to 48 hours for patients to become "therapeutic" on warfarin (as measured by increased PT/INR), so a period of overlap with heparin is needed. **Bleeding** is the most common and severe side effect; **other side effects** include GI symptoms, hemorrhagic vasculitis, urticaria, hair loss, and teratogenic effects. **Contraindications** include pregnancy (warfarin is a teratogen), liver disease, severe hypertension, tumor metastases, and active bleeding.

Epidemiology **Coumadin** is sodium warfarin and is used for **long-term anticoagulation** such as that needed in atrial fibrillation, long-term prophylaxis of DVT, arterial thrombosis, prosthetic heart valves, and recurrent pulmonary embolism.

Management Vitamin K alone if PT is increased moderately without signs of bleeding. If PT is markedly prolonged or if active bleeding is present, give fresh frozen plasma.

Complications Hemorrhage, skin necrosis, intracranial bleeding, fatal aneurysmal bleeding, hypotension during IV administration of vitamin K, and difficulty reinstating adequate anticoagulation after vitamin K use.

MINICASE 56: TRANSFUSION REACTION—HEMOLYTIC

Acute intravascular hemolysis caused by mismatches in the ABO system

- presents with fever, chills, pain at the infusion site, hypotension, and tachycardia
- positive Coombs' test, elevated BUN and creatinine, unconjugated bilirubin, hemoglobinemia, hemoglobinuria, and decreased hematocrit and serum haptoglobin
- treat by stopping transfusion, vigorous IV hydration (to maintain renal flow and filtration), and supportive care

ID/CC A **5-year-old** boy presents with **acute onset** of **high fever, noisy breathing**, and **drooling**.

HPI He had been complaining of a **sore throat**, and his parents note that his **voice was muffled**. He has **not received standard immunizations**.

PE VS: **fever** (39.4°C); tachycardia (HR 140); **tachypnea** (RR 44). PE: appears toxic with **respiratory distress** and **inspiratory stridor**; he sits with his **neck extended** and chin protruding ("SNIFFING DOG" POSITION); inspiratory retractions of chest wall, but no rales or wheezes present on lung exam; the remainder of the physical exam was deferred in order to **avoid agitating the child**.

Labs CBC: **marked leukocytosis** with left shift.

Imaging X-rays may be helpful but should be considered only in those children with minimal symptoms. Lateral neck x-ray demonstrates a swollen epiglottis obliterating the vallecula ("THUMBPRINT" SIGN).

Pathogenesis Epiglottitis can rapidly progress to total airway obstruction. ***Haemophilus influenzae*** **type B** was the most common etiologic agent until the introduction of the *H. influenzae* vaccine. *Streptococcus pneumoniae* and *Staphylococcus aureus* are other implicated agents.

Epidemiology Epiglottitis has decreased in incidence since the use of the *H. influenzae* vaccination. It usually affects children **2 to 7 years old**.

Management **Intubation** is usually required. Give **ceftriaxone** to cover *H. influenzae*; transfer to the ICU. **Do not examine the oropharynx** except in the operating room, in the presence of an anesthesiologist (risk of precipitating laryngospasm). A definitive diagnosis can be made through direct fiberoptic visualization of a cherry-red and swollen epiglottis and arytenoids.

Complications **Airway obstruction** with respiratory arrest.

Atlas Link UCVI PG-M1-087

ID/CC A 72-year-old female recovering from recent urologic surgery develops **fever, chills, lethargy**, and a **reduced urinary output** (< 30 mL/hr).

HPI Her hospital course has been otherwise unremarkable.

PE VS: **tachycardia** (HR 130); **hypotension** (BP 82/50); fever (39.6°C); tachypnea (RR 24). PE: **confused** and **disoriented; warm extremities** (due to vasodilatation in distributive shock); diffuse petechiae; no focal neurologic deficits.

Labs CBC: thrombocytopenia (due to platelet consumptive coagulopathy—**DIC**); pronounced **leukocytosis** with left shift. LFTs: hyperbilirubinemia; elevated alkaline phosphatase. Prolonged PT; elevated fibrinogen split products; BUN and creatinine elevated; $Fe_{NA} > 1\%$ (due to **acute tubular necrosis**). UA: proteinuria and tubular epithelial cell casts. ABGs: hypoxemia (due to **ARDS**); metabolic acidosis with respiratory compensation; lactic acidosis (reflects poor tissue perfusion). Blood and urine cultures grew *Escherichia coli.*

Imaging CXR: diffuse infiltrates typical of ARDS.

Pathogenesis Shock is characterized by inadequate perfusion of the tissues and may be secondary to hypovolemia, cardiac failure, massive hemorrhage, anaphylaxis, or sepsis. In septic shock, fever, chills, tachypnea, and tachycardia mark the systemic inflammatory response to the microbial invasion; when these counterregulatory mechanisms fail and dysfunction of major organ systems occurs, septic shock occurs. It is usually caused by bacteria but may also occur with fungi, mycobacteria, viruses, and protozoans.

Epidemiology The majority of cases are nosocomially acquired. Diabetes mellitus, cirrhosis, burns, vascular catheters, and immunosuppression with neutropenia predispose patients to sepsis. Localized infections in the GU tract, biliary system, or lungs may also cause bloodstream infection. The mortality of septic shock is high.

Management **IV antibiotics** and **aggressive fluid rehydration**. Admit to the ICU for hemodynamic monitoring and vasopressors. Ventilator support or hemodialysis may become necessary.

26 SHOCK—SEPTIC

Complications Complications include multiorgan dysfunction. Progressive diffuse pulmonary infiltrates and arterial hypoxemia suggest the development of **ARDS. Myocardial dysfunction** may contribute to hypotension. **Renal failure** may also occur as a result of acute tubular necrosis.

Atlas Links UCV1 M-M2-054A, M-M2-054B

MINICASE 57: CHOLERA

Caused by an exotoxin produced by *Vibrio cholerae*, activating intracellular adenylate cyclase

- presents with profuse, watery diarrhea with "rice-water" appearance
- stool exam reveals actively motile ("darting") gram-negative bacilli
- treat with oral rehydration and electrolyte and glucose repletion, tetracycline
- complications include progressive dehydration leading to hemodynamic collapse, particularly in children

MINICASE 58: PYOGENIC LIVER ABSCESS

Arises by local or hematogenous spread of bacteria from other intra-abdominal sites of infection

- presents with fever, right upper quadrant pain, and sometimes jaundice
- elevated LFTs, mass on CT and US
- treat with percutaneous drainage, broad-spectrum antibiotics

ID/CC An 18-year-old male complains of a **burning sensation during urination** and **urethral discharge**.

HPI He admits to **unprotected sex with a new sexual partner**. He denies any fevers or chills, urinary frequency, or testicular pain. He denies any new skin rash, conjunctivitis, sore throat, or arthritis.

PE VS: normal. PE: **erythema of urethral meatus**; no penile skin lesions visible; pus expressed from urethra (exudate sent for Gram stain and culture).

Labs Gram stain of urethral exudate shows **many WBCs per HPF without bacteria** (classic for chlamydial or nongonococcal urethritis); immunofluorescent slide test reveals presence of characteristic chlamydial elementary inclusions; cell culture is diagnostic.

Pathogenesis *Chlamydia trachomatis* is the most common cause of **nongonococcal** and **postgonococcal urethritis**; these terms refer, respectively, to patients with symptomatic urethritis who do not have gonococcal infection and those who become symptomatic 2 to 3 weeks after single-dose treatment for gonococcal infection. **"Postgonococcal urethritis"** is in most cases due to an untreated coexistent chlamydial infection. Other causes of nongonococcal urethritis are *Ureaplasma urealyticum*, *Trichomonas vaginalis*, and HSV.

Epidemiology *C. trachomatis* accounts for 20% to 50% of cases of symptomatic urethritis seen in heterosexual men but is less common among homosexual men. Nongonococcal urethritis is the **most common STD**. Chlamydial infection in females is often asymptomatic and is one of the leading causes of female **infertility**.

Management Empiric therapy with **azithromycin** (single dose eliminates compliance issues) or **doxycycline**. Treat pregnant women with chlamydia with erythromycin. Treat the **sexual partner** at the same time, regardless of symptoms.

Complications Complications of chlamydial STDs include PID, infertility, perihepatitis (Fitz–Hugh–Curtis syndrome), and Reiter's syndrome (in genetically predisposed HLA-B27-positive individuals).

Atlas Link UCV1 M-M2-071

27 URETHRITIS

ID/CC A 42-year-old male is brought to the emergency room after having been **stung by a bee** 20 minutes ago.

HPI The patient complains of **lightheadedness, shortness of breath,** throat tightness, and a **diffuse pruritic rash**. He was hospitalized 5 years ago after a bee sting.

PE VS: **tachycardia** (HR 120); **hypotension** (BP 90/60); **tachypnea** (RR 32). PE: alert and in mild respiratory distress; **periorbital edema and erythema** and **lingual swelling** noted; moderate **wheezes** present with slightly diminished air movement; **diffuse urticaria**.

Pathogenesis Anaphylaxis is an **IgE-mediated immediate hypersensitivity reaction** (TYPE I) that occurs in **presensitized individuals** following reexposure to an allergen. Antigen cross-links IgE on presensitized mast cells and basophils, triggering the release of vasoactive and inflammatory mediators. **Bronchospasm** and **laryngospasm** with **angioedema** may cause airway obstruction and death.

Epidemiology **Penicillins** (β-lactam antibiotics), **insect venom** (bees, wasps, hornets, fire ants), **nuts**, and **shellfish** are among the most common etiologic agents.

Management Ensure airway patency and provide supplemental **oxygen**. **Epinephrine** should be given for bronchospasm. **Antihistamines** should be given for urticaria and angioedema. **Corticosteroids** are also given but are not of immediate benefit. Consider nebulized **bronchodilators** for wheezing. Rapid infusion of large volumes of **IV crystalloids** for hypotension. IV vasopressors may be required for refractory hypotension. All patients should be admitted for **observation** and given a prescription for an epinephrine injection kit upon discharge.

Complications **Airway obstruction; cardiovascular collapse** and/or cardiac arrest. Those with preexisting cardiac disease are at risk for acute MI.

ID/CC A 20-day-old male presents with **fever, respiratory distress, decreased breast feeding**, and **lethargy**.

HPI The baby became fussy 12 hours ago. He was **delivered at 36 weeks' gestation** due to **premature rupture of the membranes** and **chorioamnionitis**.

PE VS: tachycardia (HR 174); tachypnea (RR 60); fever; Sao_2 98% on room air. PE: **ill-appearing infant** in **mild respiratory distress**; fontanelles normal; tympanic membranes normal; eyes lack luster; pupils equal, round, and reactive to light and accommodation; oral mucous membranes dry; breath sounds clear; **sternal retractions** present; decreased bowel sounds; abdomen soft and nontender; extremities with slight pallor and slightly delayed capillary refill; no rashes or petechiae.

Labs CBC: **elevated WBC** (16,000/mm^3) with **increased bands**; hemoglobin and hematocrit normal; serum bicarbonate decreased. LP: normal. UA, urine culture, and blood cultures pending.

Imaging CXR: no acute disease.

Pathogenesis Neonatal fever with sepsis can have varying presentations. Therefore, fever in neonates requires empiric antibiotic coverage and necessitates admission. Coverage for **group B streptococcus**, *Haemophilus influenzae, Meningococcus*, and ***Listeria monocytogenes*** is necessary; also investigate maternal history closely for a history of herpes. Sources to rule out immediately are CSF, urine, and chest. The finding of otitis media in an ill-appearing, febrile infant does not obviate the need for a full sepsis workup.

Epidemiology Increased incidence has been observed in **preterm** and **low-birth-weight** babies. **Perinatal complications** such as premature rupture of membranes, chorioamnionitis, **maternal PID**, fetal distress, and meconium-stained amniotic fluid have been associated with increased risk.

Management **Empiric antibiotic coverage with ampicillin and gentamicin or a cephalosporin**. Also begin fluid rehydration with crystalloid and glucose. If petechiae are present (suggestive of meningococcemia), do not wait for lumbar puncture to start antibiotic therapy. Admission to the hospital for observation is necessary.

Complications Bronchiolitis, congenital cardiac disease, and UTI.

ID/CC A 42-year-old **male** presents with the **sudden onset** of **colicky** (intermittent) right-sided **(unilateral) flank pain** that **radiates to the testicles** (labia in females).

HPI The pain is described as severe. The patient also complains of **nausea and vomiting**. He denies any history of chest pain, shortness of breath, or diarrhea. He denies any history of trauma, fever, or dysuria and was well before the pain started.

PE VS: **tachycardia** (HR 105); tachypnea (RR 22); **hypertension** (BP 160/80). PE: **diaphoretic; in severe distress; unable to find a comfortable position**; abdominal exam reveals a **soft, nondistended abdomen** with normal bowel sounds; no masses or hernias; moderate **costovertebral angle tenderness** on right side; rectal exam normal with heme-negative brown stool; GU exam normal; no evidence of testicular tenderness, masses, or hernias.

Labs UA: **hematuria** (if urine pH > 7.5, consider infection by **urea-splitting bacteria**). Urinary **crystals** may also be seen. Leukocytes suggest infection; if present, culture and sensitivity should be sent. Obtain BUN/creatinine to assess renal function.

Imaging **[A]** KUB (85% of renal stones are radiopaque; however, KUB has a low sensitivity and specificity for renal stones): a calculus is seen in the right ureter. **[B]** IVP: the "pyelogram" phase in another patient with right ureteral obstruction shows dilatation of the calyces and renal pelvis. **[C]** KUB: a different case in which bilateral staghorn calculi are seen in the pelvis of each kidney.

Pathogenesis Stones are formed when the urine is **supersaturated** with a particular mineral. **Most kidney stones (75%) are calcium salts of oxalate and phosphate**. States associated with **elevated serum calcium** levels (neoplasm, hyperparathyroidism, myeloma or sarcoidosis), hyperuricosuria, familial hypercalciuria, and renal tubular acidosis predispose the patient to renal stones. Approximately 15% of stones are **struvite** (magnesium-ammonium-phosphate) and result from chronic UTI by **urea-splitting bacteria** such as *Proteus*. The remainder are mostly **uric acid** stones resulting from gout and myeloproliferative diseases. The most common sites of **obstruction** due to renal stones **are the ureterovesical junction** and **renal pelvis**.

Epidemiology Patients are typically **adult males**. The highest incidence of renal stones is during the summer months, when **dehydration** is more likely. There is a **familial predisposition**. Oxalate-rich fresh vegetables also contribute to stone formation.

Management Hydration with IV normal saline, analgesia with a combination of narcotics and NSAIDs, and antiemetics. **Admission is required** for patients with **uncontrolled pain or intractable vomiting**, with stones > 5 mm, **with evidence of infection** (e.g., fever or leukocytes on UA), or with a **single kidney**. Stones < 5 mm that are located in the distal ureter have a high likelihood of spontaneous passage; these patients may be discharged with **pain medication** and referred to a **urologist** for follow-up.

Complications The presence of **infection** in an obstructed collecting system can quickly lead to **abscess formation, sepsis, and kidney destruction**. Prompt urologic consultation should be obtained and **antibiotics** administered. **Surgical drainage** may be required.

Atlas Link PG-A-047

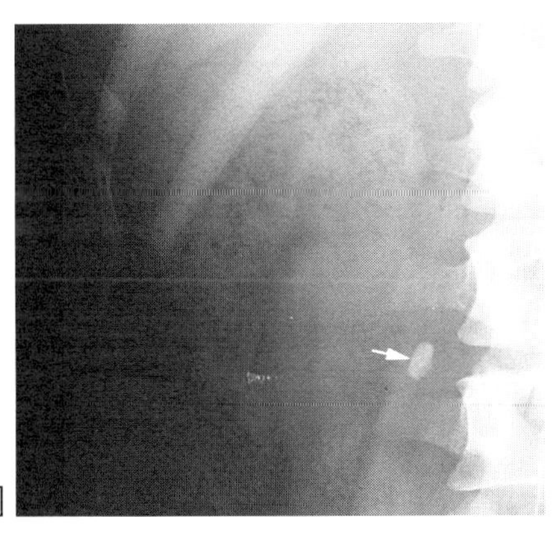

[A]

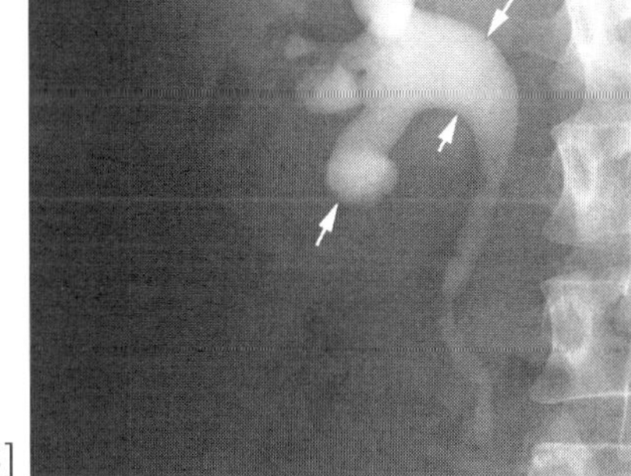

[B]

[C]

ID/CC A 30-year-old **female** presents with 3 days of progressive **flank pain, urinary frequency**, and burning sensation during urination (DYSURIA) as well as **fevers and shaking chills**.

HPI The patient is mildly **nauseated** but has not vomited and has no abdominal pain, diarrhea, or vaginal discharge. She has no history of STDs, and her last menstrual period was 2 weeks ago. She had a **UTI 3 months ago**, for which she was treated with unspecified antibiotics for 5 days.

PE VS: **fever** (38.7°C); tachycardia (HR 108). PE: in mild discomfort; sclerae anicteric; mucous membranes slightly dry; abdomen soft and nontender without rebound or guarding; **left costovertebral angle tenderness**; pelvic exam reveals scant, clear discharge; no cervical motion tenderness, no adnexal tenderness.

Labs CBC: **leukocytosis** (17,300) **with 84% neutrophils.** UA: **38 WBCs per HPF** (> 10 is significant); **abundant bacteria; leukocyte esterase and nitrites positive; WBC casts**; 5 to 10 RBCs; urine culture sent; urine pregnancy test negative.

Imaging An imaging study (either ultrasound or CT) of the kidneys should be performed if obstructive uropathy or papillary necrosis is suspected or if the patient fails to improve after 48 hours of antibiotics.

Pathogenesis Pyelonephritis usually results from an **ascending** lower UTI. It is most commonly caused by gram-negative enterobacteria, especially ***Escherichia coli***, but may also be caused by *Staphylococcus* and *Pseudomonas*. Nosocomial UTI is very common.

Epidemiology UTIs are **much more common in females**. Predisposing factors include indwelling urinary catheters, diabetes, urogenital structural abnormalities, nephrolithiasis, incomplete bladder emptying (neurogenic bladder, prostatic hypertrophy), vesicoureteral reflux, and urethral strictures. UTIs are also associated with fecal bacteria contamination during stool wiping and with diaphragm and spermicide use. Incidence is higher during pregnancy.

Management Outpatient treatment with oral antibiotics (usually 14 days of a fluoroquinolone) for stable patients who can tolerate oral fluids. Toxic-appearing patients, as well as diabetics, the elderly, and immune-compromised patients, require inpatient treatment (IV fluoroquinolone or ampicillin with gentamicin). Recurrent UTIs may be caused by structural abnormalities of the GU tract

31 PYELONEPHRITIS—ACUTE

and must be evaluated. Long-term antibiotic prophylaxis may be needed in the event of recurrent disease with no proven anatomic abnormality.

Complications Urosepsis, perinephric abscess, and acute papillary necrosis.

Atlas Links PG-M2-086A, PG-M2-086B

MINICASE 59: ACUTE RENAL FAILURE—PRERENAL

The most common presentation of acute renal failure

- caused by hypoperfusion of the kidney (dehydration, shock, decreased cardiac output), reversible
- presents with oliguria and signs of hypovolemia
- high urinary sodium and high urine specific gravity
- BUN increased more than creatinine, $Fe_{Na} < 1\%$
- treat with IV fluids, treat the underlying cause of dehydration
- may progress to acute tubular necrosis

MINICASE 60: RHABDOMYOLYSIS

Destruction of striated muscle due to several causes, including crush injuries or heat stroke

- presents with muscle pain and passage of dark brown urine, markedly increased serum BUN and creatinine, hyperkalemia, increased serum CK, and myoglobinuria
- treat with urinary alkalinization, rehydration, and mannitol
- may cause renal failure

MINICASE 61: NURSEMAID'S ELBOW

Characterized by slippage of the head of the radius beneath the annular ligament when axial traction is applied to an extended and pronated forearm

- predisposing factors include weak distal attachment of the ligament and oval shape of the proximal radius
- examination reveals a child refusing to use the arm, with forearm extended and pronated and point tenderness at the radial head
- x-rays reveal the disarticulation
- treatment involves manual closed reduction
- permanent injury seldom results, and the frequency of the disorder decreases with increasing age

ID/CC A **12-year-old boy** presents with **acute-onset**, severe right inguinal and **scrotal pain** along with **nausea and vomiting**.

HPI The child had been sleeping when the pain suddenly began. He was recently well and reports no fever, chills, diarrhea, increased urinary frequency, or dysuria. He denies any sexual activity.

PE VS: normal. PE: in moderate discomfort; holding his scrotum; abdomen soft and nontender with no guarding or rebound; normal bowel sounds present; right hemiscrotum **swollen**, erythematous, and **diffusely tender**; it is not possible to palpate the testis separate from the epididymis; right **cremasteric reflex is absent** (nonspecific); **contralateral testis has a horizontal lie** and is nontender.

Labs UA: negative.

Imaging US, testes (color doppler): to evaluate blood flow.

Pathogenesis Torsion of the spermatic cord, also known as testicular torsion, is usually associated with a **developmental defect**. The tunica vaginalis normally envelops the testes and fixes them to the posterior scrotal wall; failurc of this anchoring leaves the testes free to rotate within the scrotal sac and impinge on their blood supply, causing **ischemia** and possibly **infarction**. Patients may have a history of prior scrotal pain with spontaneous remission, likely representing torsion with spontaneous detorsion.

Epidemiology Most commonly seen in teenage boys. Often occurs during sleep, but may also occur after vigorous activity.

Management Attempt **manual detorsion** while waiting for the urologist to arrive. **Emergent surgical exploration** should be performed within 4 to 6 hours of pain onset for definitive diagnosis and treatment. Since the anatomic defect is usually bilateral, orchiopexy of both testes is necessary. Orchiectomy is necessary in cases of infarction.

Complications Testicular infarction and necrosis.

32 TESTICULAR TORSION

Epidemiology Patients are typically **adult males**. The highest incidence of renal stones is during the summer months, when **dehydration** is more likely. There is a **familial predisposition**. Oxalate-rich fresh vegetables also contribute to stone formation.

Management Hydration with IV normal saline, analgesia with a combination of narcotics and NSAIDs, and antiemetics. **Admission is required** for patients with **uncontrolled pain or intractable vomiting**, with stones > 5 mm, **with evidence of infection** (e.g., fever or leukocytes on UA), or with a **single kidney**. Stones < 5 mm that are located in the distal ureter have a high likelihood of spontaneous passage; these patients may be discharged with **pain medication** and referred to a **urologist** for follow-up.

Complications The presence of **infection** in an obstructed collecting system can quickly lead to **abscess formation, sepsis, and kidney destruction**. Prompt urologic consultation should be obtained and **antibiotics** administered. **Surgical drainage** may be required.

Atlas Link UCV1 PG-A-047

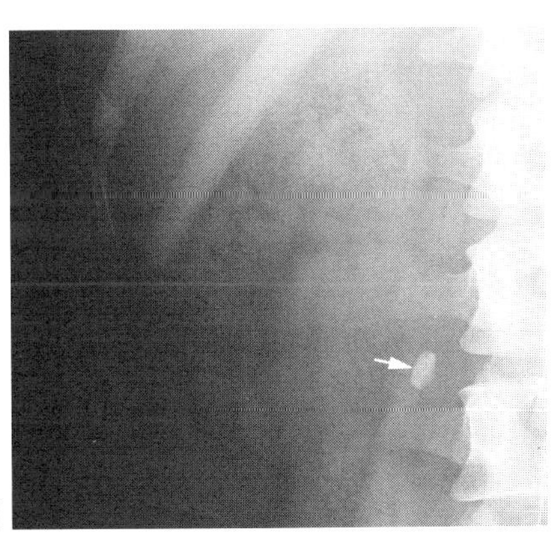

[A]

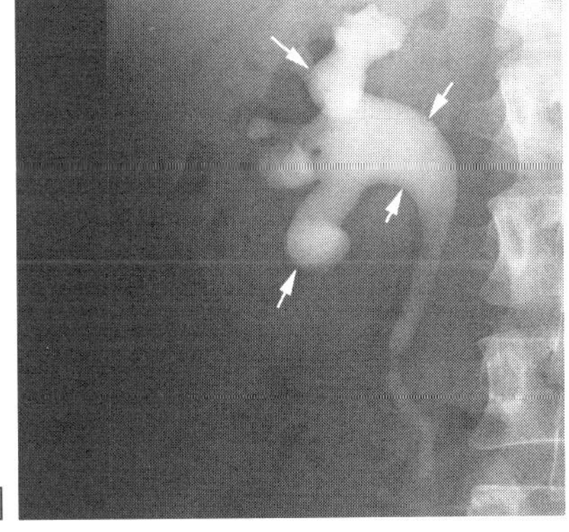

[B]

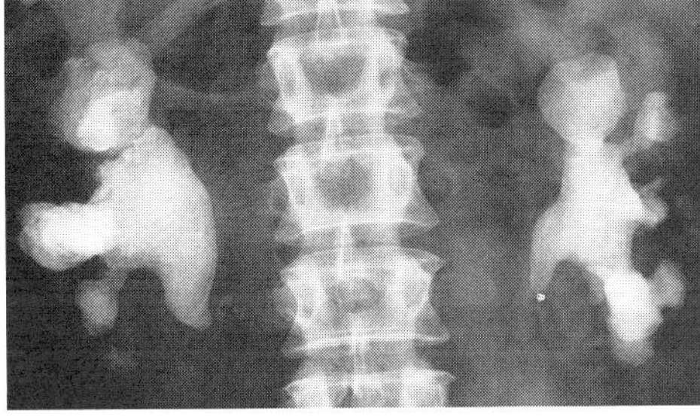

[C]

NEPHROLOGY/UROLOGY

ID/CC A 30-year-old **female** presents with 3 days of progressive **flank pain, urinary frequency**, and burning sensation during urination (DYSURIA) as well as **fevers and shaking chills**.

HPI The patient is mildly **nauseated** but has not vomited and has no abdominal pain, diarrhea, or vaginal discharge. She has no history of STDs, and her last menstrual period was 2 weeks ago. She had a **UTI 3 months ago**, for which she was treated with unspecified antibiotics for 5 days.

PE VS: **fever** (38.7°C); tachycardia (HR 108). PE: in mild discomfort; sclerae anicteric; mucous membranes slightly dry; abdomen soft and nontender without rebound or guarding; **left costovertebral angle tenderness**; pelvic exam reveals scant, clear discharge; no cervical motion tenderness, no adnexal tenderness.

Labs CBC: **leukocytosis** (17,300) **with 84% neutrophils.** UA: **38 WBCs per HPF** (> 10 is significant); **abundant bacteria; leukocyte esterase and nitrites positive; WBC casts**; 5 to 10 RBCs; urine culture sent; urine pregnancy test negative.

Imaging An imaging study (either ultrasound or CT) of the kidneys should be performed if obstructive uropathy or papillary necrosis is suspected or if the patient fails to improve after 48 hours of antibiotics.

Pathogenesis Pyelonephritis usually results from an **ascending** lower UTI. It is most commonly caused by gram-negative enterobacteria, especially ***Escherichia coli***, but may also be caused by *Staphylococcus* and *Pseudomonas*. Nosocomial UTI is very common.

Epidemiology UTIs are **much more common in females**. Predisposing factors include indwelling urinary catheters, diabetes, urogenital structural abnormalities, nephrolithiasis, incomplete bladder emptying (neurogenic bladder, prostatic hypertrophy), vesicoureteral reflux, and urethral strictures. UTIs are also associated with fecal bacteria contamination during stool wiping and with diaphragm and spermicide use. Incidence is higher during pregnancy.

Management Outpatient treatment with oral antibiotics (usually 14 days of a fluoroquinolone) for stable patients who can tolerate oral fluids. Toxic-appearing patients, as well as diabetics, the elderly, and immune-compromised patients, require inpatient treatment (IV fluoroquinolone or ampicillin with gentamicin). Recurrent UTIs may be caused by structural abnormalities of the GU tract

31 PYELONEPHRITIS—ACUTE

and must be evaluated. Long-term antibiotic prophylaxis may be needed in the event of recurrent disease with no proven anatomic abnormality.

Complications Urosepsis, perinephric abscess, and acute papillary necrosis.

Atlas Links PG-M2-086A, PG-M2-086B

MINICASE 59: ACUTE RENAL FAILURE—PRERENAL

The most common presentation of acute renal failure

- caused by hypoperfusion of the kidney (dehydration, shock, decreased cardiac output), reversible
- presents with oliguria and signs of hypovolemia
- high urinary sodium and high urine specific gravity
- BUN increased more than creatinine, $Fe_{Na} < 1\%$
- treat with IV fluids, treat the underlying cause of dehydration
- may progress to acute tubular necrosis

MINICASE 60: RHABDOMYOLYSIS

Destruction of striated muscle due to several causes, including crush injuries or heat stroke

- presents with muscle pain and passage of dark brown urine, markedly increased serum BUN and creatinine, hyperkalemia, increased serum CK, and myoglobinuria
- treat with urinary alkalinization, rehydration, and mannitol
- may cause renal failure

MINICASE 61: NURSEMAID'S ELBOW

Characterized by slippage of the head of the radius beneath the annular ligament when axial traction is applied to an extended and pronated forearm

- predisposing factors include weak distal attachment of the ligament and oval shape of the proximal radius
- examination reveals a child refusing to use the arm, with forearm extended and pronated and point tenderness at the radial head
- x-rays reveal the disarticulation
- treatment involves manual closed reduction
- permanent injury seldom results, and the frequency of the disorder decreases with increasing age

ID/CC A **12-year-old boy** presents with **acute-onset**, severe right inguinal and **scrotal pain** along with **nausea and vomiting**.

HPI The child had been sleeping when the pain suddenly began. He was recently well and reports no fever, chills, diarrhea, increased urinary frequency, or dysuria. He denies any sexual activity.

PE VS: normal. PE: in moderate discomfort; holding his scrotum; abdomen soft and nontender with no guarding or rebound; normal bowel sounds present; right hemiscrotum **swollen**, erythematous, and **diffusely tender**; it is not possible to palpate the testis separate from the epididymis; right **cremasteric reflex is absent** (nonspecific); **contralateral testis has a horizontal lie** and is nontender.

Labs UA: negative.

Imaging US, testes (color doppler): to evaluate blood flow.

Pathogenesis Torsion of the spermatic cord, also known as testicular torsion, is usually associated with a **developmental defect**. The tunica vaginalis normally envelops the testes and fixes them to the posterior scrotal wall; failure of this anchoring leaves the testes free to rotate within the scrotal sac and impinge on their blood supply, causing **ischemia** and possibly **infarction**. Patients may have a history of prior scrotal pain with spontaneous remission, likely representing torsion with spontaneous detorsion.

Epidemiology Most commonly seen in teenage boys. Often occurs during sleep, but may also occur after vigorous activity.

Management Attempt **manual detorsion** while waiting for the urologist to arrive. **Emergent surgical exploration** should be performed within 4 to 6 hours of pain onset for definitive diagnosis and treatment. Since the anatomic defect is usually bilateral, orchiopexy of both testes is necessary. Orchiectomy is necessary in cases of infarction.

Complications Testicular infarction and necrosis.

ID/CC A 76-year-old male presents with sudden-onset **low back pain** that worsens when he lies down and awakens him from sleep.

HPI The **pain radiates to the back of his thigh and leg**, is sharp, and increases on lying supine, coughing, and straining. He also has weakness and numbness of the legs. He has **advanced prostate cancer** with **metastases to the vertebral bodies** of the lumbar spine. He also notes the recent onset of **bowel and bladder incontinence**.

PE VS: normal. PE: alert and oriented ×3; muscle wasting; no jaundice or cyanosis; pallor of skin and mucous membranes; no abnormal movements; **tenderness elicited on percussion over L3–L4 vertebrae**; anesthesia from L2 downward; diminished DTRs; muscular hypotonia; strength in both legs 2/5; rectal tone decreased.

Labs LP: increased protein concentration in CSF with no concomitant increase in WBCs; normal glucose level. LFTs: alkaline phosphatase elevated (due to bone metastases).

Imaging XR, spine: **osteoblastic lesions** with pathologic **fracture of L4**. Nuc: bone scan positive. **[A]** MR, spine (gold standard for cord

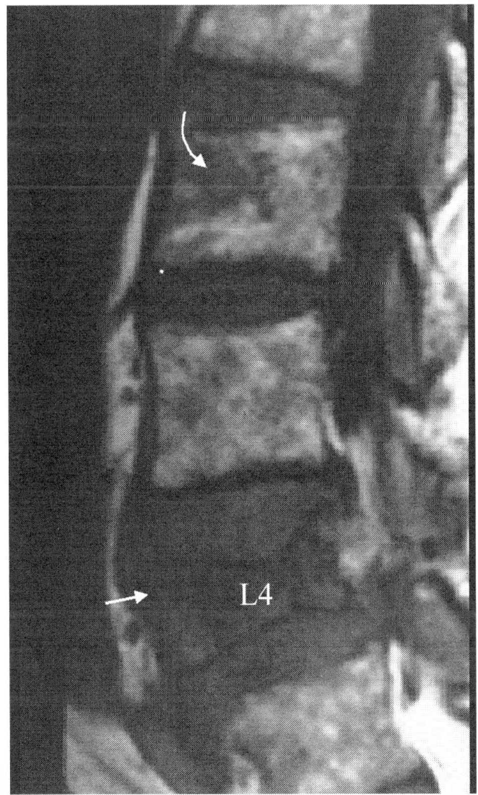

[A]

compression): **metastases** with partial collapse of L4 and probable nerve root compression.

Pathogenesis Cord compression and pathologic vertebral fractures may be due to **metastatic spread** from primary malignancies in the prostate, breast, or lung as well as from myelomas and lymphomas. Metastatic melanoma, meningiomas, and neurofibromas may also cause compression.

Management Immediate **radiation therapy** and high-dose **steroids. Surgery** for decompression.

Complications Irreversible damage to cord.

ID/CC A 24-year-old male presents with **continued generalized tonic-clonic seizure** activity for the last **30 minutes**.

HPI He has had a **history of seizures** after suffering **a severe head injury** 2 years ago; his recent history is significant only for a "head cold." He has no fever, chills, or sweats and has suffered no recent trauma. Urinary incontinence is evident. Medications include phenytoin and gabapentin.

PE VS: tachycardia (HR 122); hypertension (BP 180/110); tachypnea (RR 30). PE: well developed and well nourished without evidence of trauma; generalized tonic-clonic activity with sonorous respirations; eyes deviated toward right; pupils equal and reactive to light; no meningismus; oral bleeding from bite on tongue.

Labs Glucose normal; **phenytoin level subtherapeutic**. CBC/Lytes: normal. Calcium and magnesium normal; EtOH negative; toxicology screen negative.

Imaging CT, head (no contrast): normal.

Pathogenesis Status epilepticus is defined as multiple seizures occurring **without an intervening return to baseline consciousness**. The most common causes of status epilepticus are anticonvulsant withdrawal or noncompliance, metabolic disturbances, drug toxicity, CNS infection, CNS tumors, refractory epilepsy, and head trauma.

Epidemiology Most adults experience status epilepticus as a result of CNS pathology, drug withdrawal, or metabolic abnormalities; in 50% of children with status epilepticus, the cause is unknown.

Management Aggressive **airway maintenance** and supplemental oxygen with continuous pulse oximetry and cardiac monitoring. Control seizure activity with **benzodiazepines** such as diazepam or lorazepam; treat unresponsive cases with phenytoin or phenobarbital. Anesthesia and mechanical ventilation may be required for seizure activity that remains unresponsive.

Complications CNS injury, hyponatremia, sepsis, and substance withdrawal.

ID/CC A 57-year-old male is brought to the emergency room by paramedics after being **found unconscious** in a deserted alley; he has a **scalp laceration** with local swelling.

HPI He is a known **alcoholic** who is often brought to the emergency room by the police for public intoxication.

PE VS: bradycardia (HR 60); mild hypertension (BP 160/94); tachypnea with stertorous breathing. PE: disheveled and smells of alcohol; somnolent and responds only to deeply painful stimuli; 6-cm scalp laceration over left occiput with underlying hematoma; left pupil is 7 mm and sluggishly reactive, while right pupil is 3 mm (left dilation indicating uncal herniation); patient demonstrates decorticate posturing (flexion of arms with extended legs); normal rectal tone; Babinski's (extensor plantar reflex) present on left; no other trauma present.

Labs CBC/Lytes: normal. Glucose, BUN/creatinine, and PT/PTT normal.

Imaging CT, head: **hyperdense crescentic extra-axial fluid collection with midline shift** (ACUTE). (A hypodense fluid collection with thick membranes would be indicative of a chronic subdural hematoma.)

Pathogenesis Subdural hematoma is an accumulation of blood between the dura and arachnoid due to disruption of the **bridging veins** that connect the cerebral cortex to the **dural sinuses**. The mechanism of injury may be a direct blow or a decelerating force that tears veins. The hematoma displaces brain structures and may contribute to herniation; symptomatology may be minimal after trauma or may cause rapid death. Subdural hematomas may be divided into acute, subacute, and chronic forms. **Acute subdural hematomas** present in the first 24 hours after injury with a clinical picture of severe neurologic damage; bleeding is venous (vs. epidural hematomas). **Subacute subdural hematomas** present between 1 day and 2 weeks following injury; progressive headache is a common symptom, and there are usually focal neurologic signs. **Chronic subdural hematomas** are seen more frequently in small infants and elderly patients. They may follow trivial injuries to the head, are commonly bilateral, and occur 2 to 6 weeks after the injury; symptoms may include headache; balance difficulties or frequent falls; and confusion, seizures, or hemiparesis. MRI is better than CT for identifying a chronic subdural hematoma, since with chronicity the clot becomes isodense with brain tissue and may not be appreciated on a CT.

Epidemiology Subdural hematomas are the **most common intracranial mass lesions** that result **from trauma** to the head. Patients with acute subdural hematoma have a 50% mortality rate. The incidence of subdural hematoma increases with age (due to atrophy), anticoagulant use (mostly the subacute type), and alcoholism (due to frequent falls and atrophy).

Management Intubate immediately and hyperventilate (to prevent cerebral vasodilation); load with phenytoin (to prevent seizures). Administer mannitol (to treat cerebral edema) and place the patient in reverse Trendelenburg position. **Surgical evacuation of the hematoma** is the mainstay of treatment.

Complications Damage to the CNS may persist after surgical evacuation owing to the severe brain injury usually associated with a subdural hematoma. Other complications include increased ICP with **herniation** and post-traumatic **epilepsy**.

Atlas Link UCV1 PG-P3-032

ID/CC A 68-year-old man presents with a 20-minute episode of **dysarthria** (slurred speech), **right facial drooping and numbness**, and **right-handed weakness**.

HPI The patient's daughter claims that her father suddenly appeared "dazed" before the onset of his attack. The symptoms have **completely resolved** by the time he reaches the ER. He also reports several prior episodes of sudden, transient, mono-ocular (often left-sided) blindness (AMAUROSIS FUGAX), described as a **"shade being pulled down."** He denies any headache, vertigo, recent falls, or fever. He has a history of **hypertension** and **non-insulin-dependent diabetes** (NIDDM) and **smokes** heavily.

PE VS: no fever; hypertension (BP 145/90); normal HR; normal RR. PE: alert and comfortable; neck supple; **bruit** in left **carotid artery**; chest clear; regular rate and rhythm with no murmurs, rubs, or gallops; CN II-XII intact; language comprehension is normal and speech is fluent; able to name objects well and has normal repetition; no cerebellar signs; normal gait.

Labs CBC/Lytes: normal. Glucose elevated. ECG: normal sinus rhythm; moderate LVH (important to check ECG to rule out atrial fibrillation, a source of cerebral emboli from mural thrombi).

Imaging If the patient is having continued neurologic symptoms, a non-contrast head CT is warranted to rule out acute ischemic versus hemorrhagic stroke. Although not emergently warranted, carotid doppler ultrasound should be done to check for **carotid stenosis**, especially in light of this patient's carotid bruit. An echocardiogram should also be considered if the patient has recurrent transient ischemic attacks (TIAs) or a history of atrial fibrillation or valvular disease.

Pathogenesis Transient ischemic attacks represent **acute-onset focal** cerebrovascular dysfunction, usually lasting a few minutes to half an hour. Symptoms must resolve completely in **< 24 hours**, leaving no permanent neurologic deficits. TIAs are usually caused by embolic phenomena, often dislodged from an extracranial artery or from the heart (due to mural thrombus, atrial fibrillation, mitral valve disease, infective endocarditis, or prosthetic valves). **Carotid disease** usually presents with **unilateral** symptoms such as paresthesias, sensory loss, weakness, or paralysis in the face, hands, and limbs; language disturbance such as aphasia and dysarthria; and visual loss in the eye contralateral to the affected limbs. **Vertebrobasilar involvement** presents as vertigo, ataxic gait, bilateral visual disturbances, diplopia, drop attacks, hemiparesis, paresthesias, and dysarthria.

Epidemiology Stroke is a leading cause of death in the United States, and TIAs are the **most common predictor of a subsequent stroke**. Patients with TIA are often evaluated by their physician once the symptoms have already subsided, so neurologic signs are generally not seen. **Risk factors** include prior embolic phenomena, **hypertension, diabetes mellitus, CAD, smoking**, OCP use, **atherosclerosis, atrial fibrillation**, and dilated cardiomyopathy.

Management Give glucose if the patient is hypoglycemic. Rule out evolving stroke in patients with persistent neurologic symptoms. Patients with escalating frequency of TIAs may need admission for **acute anticoagulation** with heparin; asymptomatic patients may be admitted for further workup or sent home on **aspirin** or **ticlopidine** (to reduce the risk of stroke) and evaluated as outpatients. **Carotid endarterectomy** is recommended for high-grade (> 70%) stenosis in accessible locations; the best results are obtained if performed early after TIA. Those with inoperable carotid lesions or emboli of cardiac origin may require **long-term anticoagulation** with warfarin.

Complications Progression to **stroke**.

ID/CC A 21-year-old female presents with **acute-onset** right **lower quadrant pain**, nausea, and vomiting.

HPI The patient has no fever or chills, denies increased urinary frequency or dysuria, and has no vaginal bleeding, diarrhea, or constipation. She has been sexually active for 4 years but has never taken OCPs (OCPs suppress the growth of ovarian cysts), and her last menstrual period occurred regularly. She has no history of STDs.

PE VS: normal. PE: in mild discomfort; abdomen is **tender to palpation** in right lower quadrant with no palpable masses; **moderate voluntary guarding**; no rebound tenderness; normal active bowel sounds; pelvic exam discloses no cervical motion tenderness or discharge; **tender mass in right adnexa**; rectal exam nontender with heme-negative brown stool.

Labs CBC/UA: normal. Urine pregnancy test negative.

Imaging US: cystic right adnexal mass.

Pathogenesis The growth of an ovarian cyst is accompanied by elongation of the pedicle and by an increase in weight, predisposing the cyst to **twisting** (TORSION), which compromises the vascular supply, causing ischemia and possible infarction. The torsion may be partial or complete, and the cyst may be benign (e.g., serous or mucinous cystadenoma) or malignant (e.g., serous cystadenocarcinoma). Small cysts (which have a short pedicle) and very large cysts (which are fixed and cannot turn) do not usually undergo torsion.

Epidemiology The **right ovary is more frequently twisted** than the left one, and there is a greater frequency of torsion during pregnancy and in children.

Management Emergency laparoscopy or laparotomy with ovarian or adnexal detorsion or removal; IV fluids to maintain hemodynamic stability.

Complications **Shock; ovarian necrosis**.

ID/CC A 24-year-old female presents with vaginal bleeding **10 weeks** into her first pregnancy.

HPI She has soaked two pads in the last 2 hours and has been having mild intermittent abdominal cramps throughout the day. She describes blood clots in the pads but no fetal tissue. She denies having any lightheadedness or dizziness with postural changes and also denies any fever, chills, sweats, or abdominal trauma. She is taking prenatal vitamins and has no known drug allergies; **maternal blood type is O negative**.

PE VS: normal. PE: well-appearing female; normal active bowel sounds; abdomen soft, nontender, and nondistended; blood and clots in pelvic vaginal vault; **cervical os closed** to cotton applicator; no fetal tissue visible; no adnexal tenderness and no mass palpable; no cervical motion tenderness.

Labs CBC: normal.

Imaging US, transvaginal: confirms intrauterine pregnancy.

Pathogenesis **Threatened abortion** presents with vaginal bleeding and mild cramps, but the **os is closed** and no fetal tissue has been lost. There is, however, a danger of progression to abortion. **Inevitable abortion** implies that the abortion is unavoidable and presents with profuse vaginal bleeding and an **open cervical os** on pelvic exam.

Epidemiology Vaginal bleeding in the first trimester has an incidence of 25%. Of these, about half will suffer a loss of the pregnancy. A strong predictor of spontaneous abortion is a history of a previous episode. First-trimester bleeding is not always pathologic.

Management IV fluids if vital signs are unstable or the patient is symptomatic. **Transvaginal ultrasound** to rule out an ectopic pregnancy. If the mother is Rh negative, she should receive **RhoGAM** to protect her against isoimmunization from fetal-maternal transmission. Hemodynamic stability must be monitored and supported if bleeding is severe.

Complications Complications of abortion include missed abortion and DIC; incomplete abortion and sepsis; hydatidiform mole; and invasive choriocarcinoma.

ABORTION—THREATENED

ID/CC A 23-year-old male college student is brought to the ER by his roommate because of marked **restlessness** and **euphoria** as well as **anxiety** and **paranoia**.

HPI The roommate states that the patient rarely sleeps **(insomnia)**, barely eats **(anorexia)**, and has **lost weight**. He has seen the patient smoke **"ice"** for the past several days.

PE VS: **hypertension** (BP 165/100); **tachycardia** (HR 123); **fever** (38.8°C); normal RR. PE: **sweaty, agitated**, and **anxious; pupils dilated** (MYDRIASIS); neck supple without meningismus; chest clear to auscultation; cardiac exam tachycardic but otherwise unremarkable; abdomen soft with active bowel sounds; patient is paranoid and intermittently combative; **hyperreflexia** (increased DTRs) is present.

Labs CBC/Lytes: normal. BUN and creatinine normal. UA: **toxicology screen positive for amphetamines**. ECG (to rule out arrhythmias or ischemia): sinus tachycardia; no ischemic changes; TFTs normal. **Check for elevated CPK and myoglobinuria**, which will be present in rhabdomyolysis.

Imaging Head CT is indicated in the presence of focal neurologic deficits, decreased level of consciousness, or suspected intracerebral hemorrhage.

Pathogenesis Amphetamines (also known as "speed," "crank," "ice," or "crystal meth") may be taken by the oral, IV, or inhalation route. They are abused primarily for their **euphoric** and **stimulatory** effects. Clinically they are used for the treatment of attention-deficit disorder, narcolepsy, and weight reduction.

Epidemiology Amphetamine abuse is often accompanied by alcohol ingestion or benzodiazepine abuse (to counteract the dysphoric effects).

Management Ensure airway protection first. Patients should be placed on a cardiac monitor and may require ICU admission. Treat agitation and seizures with **benzodiazepines**. Severe hypertension may require vasodilators such as **nitroprusside** (to prevent intracerebral hemorrhage). Use **beta-blockers** such as propranolol for tachyarrhythmias. Treat hyperthermia with **antipyretics** and external cooling if necessary. **Hemodialysis** may be necessary for rhabdomyolysis (due to hyperthermia and agitation, which can lead to severe myoglobinuria).

Complications Death due to **hyperthermia, cardiac arrhythmia**, or **intracerebral hemorrhage**. Rhabdomyolysis and seizures may also occur.

MINICASE 62: MDMA (ECSTASY) TOXICITY

An illicit "empathogenic" drug (phenylalkylamine compound 3,4-methylenedioxymethamphetamine) that on oral ingestion causes excitation of the CNS

- patients present with a euphoric mood, hallucinations (individuals' setting, expectations, and ability to cope determine response to hallucinations), and, on physical exam, pupillary dilatation, tachycardia, diaphoresis, and tremors
- diagnosis rests on history, physical evidence, and exam
- treatment includes reassurance in a structured, secure environment and benzodiazepines to decrease anxiety
- complications include accidents, prolonged psychosis, flashbacks, anxiety, and depression

ID/CC A 28-year-old anesthesiology resident is dumped in front of the ER by "friends" who quickly drive away after stating that the patient was **found unresponsive on the floor**.

HPI The patient has a **history of IV drug use**.

PE VS: **bradypnea** (RR 6); **bradycardia** (HR 50); **hypotension** (BP 90/60); mild hypothermia (36°C); Sao_2 92% on 6 L/min oxygen. PE: **stuporous** and without signs of trauma; **pinpoint pupils** (MIOSIS); **cyanotic lips**; neck supple; chest clear; cardiac exam unremarkable; abdomen nontender with **decreased bowel sounds**; needle **"track" marks** noted along arms (stigmata of chronic IV use); skin is cool with two subcutaneous abscesses.

Labs Glucose normal. UA: toxicology screen positive for opioids. Blood alcohol level increased (alcohol abuse accompanies many cases of drug abuse). ABGs may demonstrate **hypoxemia and respiratory acidosis**.

Imaging CXR: normal (rule out aspiration or pulmonary edema, or if the patient was intubated). Obtain a head CT if the patient does not respond appropriately to naloxone or if there is suspected head trauma.

Pathogenesis Heroin is a synthetic **derivative of morphine** (an opioid). It can be injected intravenously ("MAINLINING") or subcutaneously ("SKIN POPPING"), or it may be smoked or snorted. Unintentional overdoses frequently occur because of the **wide margin of purity** of heroin purchased illicitly on the street (heroin is commonly combined with quinine, which in itself has serious sequelae); inexperienced and first-time users are also at risk. Patients develop tolerance to opioids (morphine, meperidine, oxycodone, hydromorphone) and may demonstrate drug-seeking behavior.

Epidemiology Abuse is more common in **inner cities**, but its incidence is increasing among the middle class. Health professionals have a higher incidence of opiate abuse, partly because of easy access.

Management **Intubate** if there is emesis, severe respiratory compromise, or no response to naloxone. **Naloxone** (an opiate antagonist) IV or IM for respiratory depression usually induces a rapid onset of increased respiratory rate and dramatic improvement in mental status; repeated doses may be necessary since its duration of action is 1 to 2 hours. Naloxone may cause severe acute withdrawal symptoms (rhinorrhea, piloerection, yawning, diaphoresis, colicky abdominal pain, and irritability). Recreational users may become very combative and irritable, while patients with chronic pain may be thrust into severe pain.

Complications **Tolerance and opioid withdrawal** are chronic consequences of abuse. Acute complications include apnea, pulmonary edema, endocarditis, bacterial and fungal septicemia, abscess formation, HIV, and hepatitis infection. Heroin addiction and its associated cost causes complex long-term social disturbances, including **violence, crime, prostitution**, and antisocial behavior. The combined risk of these social and physical effects is a common cause of **premature death**.

ID/CC A **23-year-old male** with **schizophrenia** presents with **confusion** and **muscle rigidity** of several hours' duration and acute-onset **high fever**.

HPI The patient takes **phenothiazine** (dopaminergic-blocking antipsychotic), and his **dose was recently increased**. He had no antecedent headaches, neck pain, photophobia, or fever.

PE VS: **tachycardia** (HR 125); **hypotension** (BP 90/60); **fever** (40.2°C). PE: **appears dazed** and is **markedly diaphoretic** (autonomic instability); pupils equal and reactive; mucous membranes dry; neck stiff; no murmurs; normal active bowel sounds present; **marked rigidity of all major muscle groups** with **hyperreflexia**; no focal neurologic findings.

Labs CBC: mild leukocytosis. **Increased CPK** (muscle hyperactivity). ABGs: **metabolic acidosis**. UA: **myoglobinuria. LP: normal**.

Imaging CXR: no infiltrates.

Pathogenesis Neuroleptic malignant syndrome is a **life-threatening idiosyncratic reaction to neuroleptic agents** (phenothiazines, thioxanthenes, dibenzoxepines, and butyrophenones) that is characterized by generalized rigidity, mental status changes, autonomic instability, and high fever. The most commonly involved drug is **haloperidol**. The pathogenesis involves central dopaminergic blockade. **The diagnosis is made after excluding other possible causes** of the patient's signs and symptoms (DIAGNOSIS OF EXCLUSION).

Epidemiology Has a relatively low incidence but a **mortality rate of 20%**. A higher incidence has been noted in young men. The onset of symptoms is usually within 1 week of initiating drug therapy or changing dosage; symptoms generally last for 10 days.

Management **Discontinue the neuroleptic drug**; intubate for airway compromise or respiratory failure. **Rapid cooling** via mist and fanning (antipyretics are rarely effective) or ice if necessary. Benzodiazepines are given to decrease muscle rigidity. **Dantrolene** (relaxes skeletal muscle by inhibiting the release of calcium from the sarcoplasmic reticulum) and bromocriptine (a dopamine agonist) have been used with variable success.

Complications Death, often due to **lack of recognition** of disease entity; renal failure due to **rhabdomyolysis**; and cardiac arrhythmias.

ID/CC A 27-year-old female is brought to the ER 2 hours after taking a handful of imipramine (tricyclic antidepressant) tablets. The patient is anxious and complains of **dry mouth, blurred vision, and flushing of the face** (due to anticholinergic effect).

HPI The patient has a history of **depression** and **prior suicide attempts**. She denies any other ingestion, alcohol use, or illicit drug use.

PE VS: **fever** (38.8°C) (due to anticholinergic-induced inability to sweat); **tachycardia** (HR 125); **hypotension** (BP 90/50). PE: **confused**; intermittent **myoclonic jerks** of arms and legs noted; **dilated pupils** (MYDRIASIS); absent bowel sounds; **DTRs hyperactive**; skin warm, dry, and flushed.

Labs Toxicologic panel (especially to check acetaminophen and salicylate levels) and EtOH level. CPK normal. ECG: sinus tachycardia with premature ventricular contractions; **prolonged QRS and PR intervals**.

Imaging None necessary unless suspected aspiration or intubation necessary.

Pathogenesis Tricyclic antidepressants (TCAs) act by blocking the reuptake of norepinephrine and serotonin and are used for a range of disorders, including depression, enuresis, anxiety, and peripheral neuropathies. TCAs have significant lethal potential in the event of an overdose. The clinical presentation can vary from **anticholinergic symptoms** (agitation, delirium, dry mouth, sinus tachycardia, urinary retention, decreased peristalsis, sedation, coma) to cardiotoxicity (prolonged QRS intervals, arrhythmias, and decreased inotropy) secondary to sodium channel blockade. TCAs include secondary amines (nortriptyline, desipramine) and tertiary amines (imipramine, amitriptyline, doxepin); tertiary amines are more frequently associated with anticholinergic side effects and orthostatic hypotension than are secondary ones.

Management Intubate to protect the airway in obtunded or comatose patients; give **activated charcoal**. Gastric lavage is controversial, although it may have a role in cases of massive ingestion that present early to the ER. Give benzodiazepines for agitation and for seizures; give **sodium bicarbonate** for QRS prolongation > 100 msec, ventricular arrhythmias, or refractory hypotension. Dialysis and forced diuresis are not effective for TCA overdosage because TCAs have a large volume of distribution and are highly protein-bound. All patients with intentional ingestions will require **psychiatric evaluation** and hospitalization once medically cleared. Physostigmine may be used to reverse low-dose anticholinergic effects in those with minimal toxicity and no cardiac depression.

Complications **Seizures** (common), death due to respiratory depression, hyperpyrexia, shock, and **cardiac arrhythmias**. Secondary complications may include aspiration pneumonia, anoxic encephalopathy, and rhabdomyolysis.

ID/CC A 30-year-old female complains of a **swollen nose and black eye** that she incurred when she tripped, fell, and struck her head on an end table.

HPI She denies any loss of consciousness, visual disturbances, or alcohol consumption and reports no numbness, tingling, diplopia, loss of balance, or disturbances of gait. She has no relevant medical history and takes no medications.

PE VS: normal. PE: well developed and well nourished; tearful; skull is atraumatic; tympanic membranes bilaterally normal; pupils equal, round, and reactive to light; extraocular muscles intact; swelling and point tenderness over bridge of nose; ecchymosis along infraorbital ridge; facial bones without crepitus; nares have dried blood bilaterally with no septal hematoma; oropharynx normal; ecchymosis on medial aspect of right upper arm; back reveals several areas of **ecchymosis in various stages of resolution**.

Imaging XR: fracture of nasal bone.

Pathogenesis It is necessary to maintain a high index of suspicion for domestic violence, because many victims are reluctant to come forward. Domestic violence can take many forms, including physical, emotional, and sexual abuse.

Epidemiology Risk factors include **pregnancy**, single status, **alcohol or drug abuse**, and a **family history** of domestic violence. Some believe that up to one-third of ER visits by females with any complaint may arise from partner abuse. About 50% of women are battered at some point in their lives, one-third of them repeatedly. One-third of pregnant women are physically abused.

Management **Referral to social services**, including a shelter or safe house. Complete **documentation** such as pictures, diagrams, or, as in this case, documentation of a fractured nose by radiography is helpful. **Early intervention** is key in preventing recurrences.

43 DOMESTIC VIOLENCE

ID/CC A 28-year-old **female** student with a history of **depression** and **past suicide attempts** states, "I'm afraid I might do something to myself."

HPI The patient reports recent **social stressors** at home, expresses feelings of **hopelessness** and worthlessness, and wishes that "it would all just end." She has already purchased a bottle of acetaminophen (PLAN) and has imagined herself taking several handfuls of pills (IDEATION). She denies any ingestion yet.

PE VS: normal. PE: slightly disheveled woman with clearly **depressed affect**; tearful and apologetic for "wasting your time"; mental status exam confirms **suicidal ideation** with a definitive **plan** and the potential to act upon thoughts.

Labs No labs are necessary unless it is suspected that the patient has already taken some pills as a suicidal gesture/attempt, in which case a toxicology screen should be ordered.

Pathogenesis Suicidality is **associated with depression**. Those with increased social stressors, poor coping mechanisms, chronic diseases, and psychotic illnesses are also at risk. Alcohol is a significant factor in many suicide attempts.

Epidemiology The suicide rate in the United States is 20 per 100,000. Individuals with depression have a lifetime risk of 10% to 15%. **Males tend to be more successful** in completing suicide, but **females tend to exhibit more suicide attempts**.

Management Any person who is acutely suicidal requires **emergent inpatient hospitalization** with psychiatric evaluation. If patients refuse admission, they **must be admitted involuntarily to protect them from harming themselves**. Ensure that the patient is not left alone at any time. Patients should always be medically cleared with a physical exam and appropriate lab work if necessary before being transferred or admitted to a psychiatry service. Administer charcoal PO if any ingestion is suspected.

Complications Completion of the suicidal threat.

ID/CC A 34-year-old female complains of **difficulty breathing**.

HPI She has a history of asthma and reports 1 week of productive cough and rhinorrhea. She also describes fevers, chills, and sweats. She had **a prior intubation for an asthma exacerbation**. Medications include albuterol and flunisolide at home.

PE VS: tachycardia (HR 130), **pulsus paradoxus**; tachypnea (RR 38); fever (38.2°C); Sao_2 70% on room air. PE: well-developed, well-nourished female with **severe respiratory distress** and **mild cyanosis**; no tonsillar adenopathy or erythema; trachea is midline; absent lung sounds in bilateral posterior bases; faint expiratory **wheezing** with increased expiratory-to-inspiratory (E:I) ratio; heart tachycardic with no gallops; accessory muscles used for breathing.

Labs CBC: WBC elevated with left shift; **eosinophilia**.

Imaging CXR: right lower lobe infiltrate.

Pathogenesis Asthma is a disease of hyperreactive airway spasm and inflammation. The disease can be **extrinsic** (atopic) or **intrinsic** in nature and has an **immediate phase** and a delayed **cellular phase** (as inflammatory cells are summoned by various chemotactic factors). Patients are generally asymptomatic between attacks. A causative trigger for acute exacerbations can often be identified. In this case, the trigger is the underlying pneumonia. Other potential triggers include exercise, dust, dust mites, pollen, smoke, cold air, and certain drugs.

Epidemiology Asthma is a disease that affects about 5% of the adult population in the United States. Adult males are affected more than females; in children, the ratio is 1:1. There are about 5,000 deaths per year from asthma; this has been consistent for many years.

Management **Albuterol** and **ipratropium** bromide nebulizers and IV **corticosteroids** to reverse bronchial obstruction. Hospitalization is indicated in this case owing to the room-air hypoxia and underlying pneumonia. Community-acquired pneumonia should be treated with a macrolide antibiotic such as azithromycin or erythromycin. IV fluid replacement should also be initiated. For long-term management, patients should avoid exacerbating triggers and use **steroid inhalers** to prevent recurrent attacks.

Complications Complications of severe asthma exacerbations include tension pneumothorax, pneumomediastinum, and cardiac arrest.

ASTHMA—SEVERE ACUTE

ID/CC An 82-year-old male develops **acute-onset shortness of breath at rest** and **pleuritic chest pain**.

HPI The patient has been **recovering from hip replacement surgery** that was performed 3 days ago. He denies a history of cardiac disease.

PE VS: **tachycardia** (HR 126); hypotension (BP 72/52); **tachypnea** (RR 32); fever (38.9°C). PE: apprehensive and restless; cyanosis; localized rales and wheezes and a pleural friction **rub**; wide physiologic splitting of S_2; JVD; good peripheral pulses.

Labs CBC: leukocytosis. Elevated ESR. ECG: sinus tachycardia; right axis deviation and S_1-Q_3-$\perp_3$ (flipped T wave in III) pattern seen. ABGs: arterial hypoxemia, hypocapnia, and respiratory alkalosis; **alveolar-arterial oxygen gradient increased**.

Imaging **[A]** CXR (often normal): peripheral wedge-shaped density (HAMPTON'S HUMP) (1) indicating pulmonary infarction. **[B]** V/Q scan: a different case with multiple mismatched wedge-shaped perfusion defects. **[C]** Ventilation scan: normal. **[D]** Arteriogram, pulmonary: a different case with a large right pulmonary artery embolus.

Pathogenesis Deep venous thrombosis is promoted by **stasis, abnormalities in the vessel wall**, and **alterations in blood coagulability**. Pulmonary emboli typically arise from thrombi of the deep venous system that have propagated to above the knee. Platelets aggregate to form a white thrombus, followed by the formation of a large red thrombus; growth is then continued by deposition of fibrin and platelet accretion. Pulmonary thromboembolism (PTE) produces **intrapulmonary dead space**, i.e., regions that are ventilated but not perfused. Loss of alveolar surfactant occurs later and can result in alveolar instability, atelectasis, and arterial hypoxemia. An increase in pulmonary vascular resistance, pulmonary hypertension, acute RV failure, tachycardia, and a decrease in cardiac output may also occur. PTE may also be a cause of syncope, supraventricular tachycardia, and the sudden worsening of CHF and COPD.

Epidemiology Pulmonary thromboembolism is a leading cause of morbidity and mortality in the United States. It has been estimated that a large number of nonfatal pulmonary thromboemboli occur each year; evidence of recent or old embolism has been detected in approximately 25% of autopsies.

Management **Heparin** infusion, except in patients with a known hemostatic defect or active bleeding. Heparin prevents recurrence, promotes resolution, and inhibits the growth of thromboemboli. There are few clinical signs to predict DVT; hence, prophylaxis is the best option. Low-dose heparin and intermittent venous compression are the most effective measures. Three- to six-month warfarin therapy is indicated for a first-time event, and lifelong therapy is indicated for recurrent embolism. Pregnant women cannot take **warfarin** because of possible **teratogenic effects**. Trauma patients, whose risk factors are unknown, should receive an inferior vena caval filter to guard against embolization. Thrombolytic therapy (urokinase, streptokinase, and tPA) hastens the resolution of emboli; however, these drugs are associated with hemorrhagic risks, especially in patients who have had vascular lesions, trauma, stroke, peptic ulcer disease, angiography, or recent catheterizations. Surgical therapy is rarely considered because of poor clinical results.

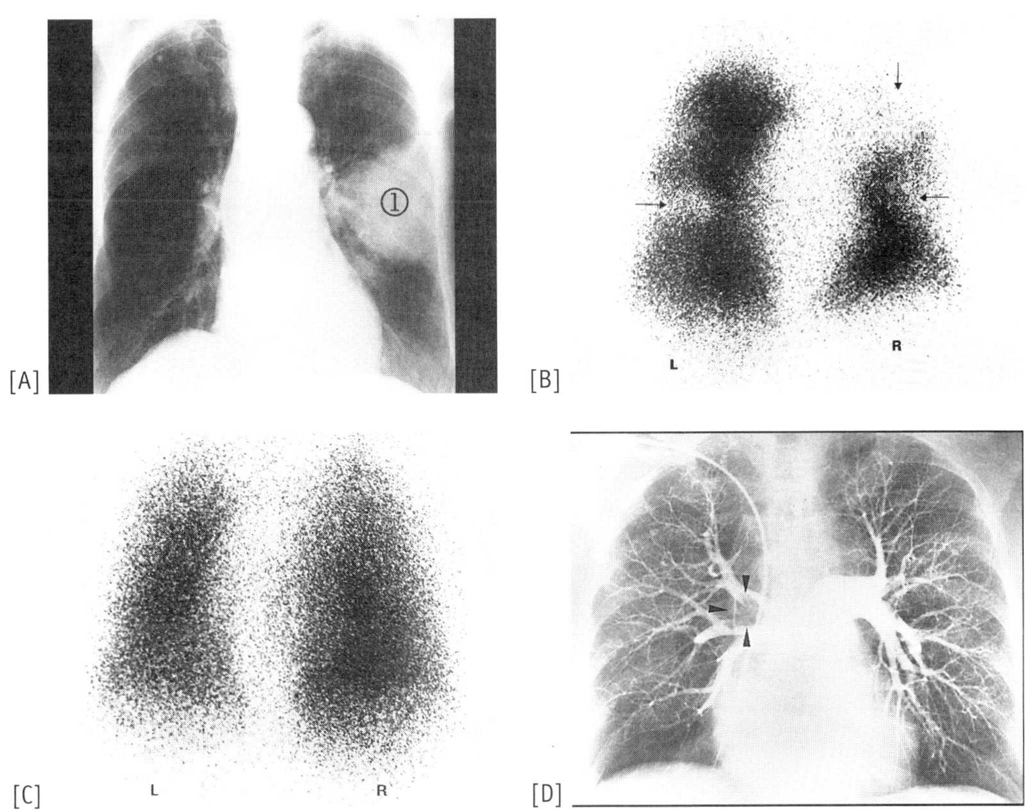

Complications Infarction of lung tissue is infrequent (affects about 10% of cases) and is increased by cardiac or pulmonary disease (CHF, mitral stenosis, or COPD). The majority of pulmonary thromboemboli resolve within the first few days. Two mechanisms promote restored blood flow: the fibrinolytic system and organization. Emboli that do not resolve could result from well-organized thrombi and deficiencies in fibrinolytic attack.

Atlas Links UCV1 PG-P2-091, PM-P2-091

MINICASE 63: FAT EMBOLISM

Embolization of fat 24 to 72 hours after fracture of long bone

- presents with petechiae (usually seen in the sclera), fever, dyspnea, cyanosis, and hypotension
- refractory hypoxemia with hypercapnia, fat in urine and sputum
- CXR with late pulmonary infiltrates
- treat with ventilatory support
- prevent by early stabilization of long-bone fractures

Atlas Link: UCV1 PM-P2-082

MINICASE 64: FLAIL CHEST

Loss of bony continuity of one segment of the chest wall caused by multiple segmental rib fractures

- presents with paradoxical movement of the chest wall
- treat with adequate chest wall stabilization, supplemental oxygen, pain control, endotracheal intubation, and mechanical ventilation if necessary

MINICASE 65: PNEUMOTHORAX—OPEN

A large defect in the chest

- usually due to a penetrating injury
- injury causes a "sucking chest wound," which is passage of air through the chest wall with inspiration
- treat with sterile dressing closing the wound on three sides, chest tube, and then surgical closure

ID/CC A 43-year-old woman presents to the emergency department with a 3-week history of periodic **headache, nausea, dizziness,** and **fatigue**.

HPI The patient initially **thought she had the flu**, but the symptoms have persisted. She notes that her **husband and children have similar symptoms**, which began around the time it started to get cold outside. The symptoms are worse in the mornings and **improve whenever she is at work** (out of the house). She reports no fevers, chills, or sweats and has had no cough, nasal congestion, or sore throat.

PE VS: normal; Sao_2 98% on room air (pulse oximetry is unreliable in carbon monoxide poisoning). PE: alert; appears nauseated but in no respiratory distress; skin is warm and dry; neurologic exam normal.

Labs **Carboxyhemoglobin** level elevated (levels often do not correlate with the severity of clinical intoxication); venous blood may appear **"cherry red."**

Pathogenesis Carbon monoxide is a colorless, odorless gas produced by the incomplete combustion of carbon-containing compounds. It binds to hemoglobin with an affinity 250 times that of oxygen, resulting in **decreased oxygen-carrying capacity** and **impaired oxygen delivery** to tissues (oxyhemoglobin curve shifts to the left). Exposure occurs from furnaces, portable kerosene **heaters**, stoves, barbecues, **automobile exhaust**, and **fires**. Chronic exposure will present with **vague** and nonspecific **flulike symptoms**, while severe acute poisoning may result in **seizures** or **coma**.

Epidemiology Carbon monoxide is a **leading cause of poisoning morbidity and mortality**. It is often seen in the **winter**, when heaters are used and windows are sealed, decreasing ventilation. The diagnosis is frequently missed, since the symptoms are nonspecific.

Management Maintain airway, and intubate if comatose. Oxygen is the mainstay of treatment. Give **100% oxygen by face mask** (reduces the half-life of carboxyhemoglobin from 5 hours to 1 hour). **Hyperbaric oxygen** should be considered for patients with severe intoxication or pregnant patients who either are symptomatic or have a carboxyhemoglobin level > 20.

47 CARBON MONOXIDE POISONING

Complications Delayed neurologic sequelae include **memory difficulties, personality changes**, parkinsonism, and persistent vegetative state.

MINICASE 66: CAUSTIC INGESTION

Commonly ingested caustic substances (cleaning products, battery liquid, rust removers, and bleach) severely injure the squamous epithelial cells of the oropharynx, hypopharynx, and esophagus

- alkaline substances cause a liquefactive necrosis, whereas acid causes coagulation necrosis
- the severity of damage depends on pH, concentration, volume, and duration of contact
- presents with dyspnea, dysphagia, abdominal pain, nausea, and vomiting, with physical examination showing signs of airway obstruction, burns, or acute abdomen
- CXR may show mediastinitis, pneumoperitoneum, and aspiration pneumonitis
- treat by dilution with water or milk and avoiding emesis
- complications include hemorrhage, delayed airway obstruction, perforation, strictures, and squamous cell carcinoma

MINICASE 67: CYANIDE POISONING

Acquired from shoe polish, metal plating, or fumigation chemicals

- causes inhibition of cytochrome oxidase, which is involved in electron transport
- presents with vertigo, dyspnea, nausea, vomiting, and classic bitter almond scent on breath, developing into convulsions, respiratory failure, and cardiac arrhythmias
- treat with sodium nitrite and sodium thiosulfate, intubate if necessary
- complications include death

MINICASE 68: ETHYLENE GLYCOL INGESTION

Ethylene glycol is found in antifreeze

- presents with nausea, vomiting, ataxia, and obtundation, leading to seizures and acute respiratory distress syndrome
- increased anion-gap metabolic acidosis, positive ethylene glycol blood levels, and oxalate crystals in urine
- treat with ethanol drip, alkalinize urine with sodium bicarbonate, intubate if necessary, hemodialysis if necessary
- complications include cardiovascular collapse and renal failure

ID/CC A 25-year-old man is found in a **stuporous state**.

HPI For the past hour the patient has been complaining of severe **headache**, giddiness, and **blurring of vision**; a few hours before, he had consumed **bootleg liquor**. He is an alcoholic.

PE VS: **tachypnea**. PE: drowsy and in moderate respiratory distress; breath smells of alcohol; funduscopy reveals blurring of edges of disks and diminished size of arterial and venous vessels.

Labs ABGs: severe **metabolic acidosis** with increased anion and osmolar gap and low lactate levels. Serum methanol levels markedly elevated.

Pathogenesis The toxic metabolites of methanol—formic acid and formaldehyde—are responsible for producing both metabolic acidosis and optic neuritis. The **severity of acidosis** is a **better predictor of outcome** than serum methanol levels. There are signs of primary optic atrophy with degeneration of ganglion cells in the retina.

Epidemiology Ethanol is frequently ingested along with other drugs, both in suicide attempts and in recreational drug abuse. Often ingested as substitutes for ethanol, ethylene glycol (antifreeze) and methanol (wood alcohol) can cause profound and often fatal poisoning.

Management Hemodialysis for high serum levels of methanol; **IV ethanol** blocks the metabolism of methanol to toxic metabolites. Give sodium bicarbonate to counter acidosis; vitamin B_{12} may minimize visual loss.

Complications If the patient survives, vision may rapidly decline, passing through stages of contracted fields and absolute central scotomata to blindness.

ID/CC A 4-year-old girl is brought to the emergency department with acute-onset abdominal pain with **emesis, tinnitus**, and **fever**.

HPI She had been found 6 hours earlier drinking from a bottle of **oil of wintergreen** (METHYL SALICYLATE). She is an otherwise-healthy child and is up to date with her vaccinations.

PE VS: **fever** (39.3°C); **tachypnea** (RR 36) with **hyperpnea** (increase in depth of respiration; the most common presenting sign); hypotension (BP 100/60). PE: sleepy; mucous membranes dry **(dehydration)**; chest clear; abdomen diffusely tender without rebound; active bowel sounds present; **marked diaphoresis**.

Labs Lytes: **hypokalemia; increased anion gap**. ABGs: **mixed metabolic acidosis** with **respiratory alkalosis. Serum salicylate increased 6 hours post-ingestion**.

Imaging None necessary unless aspiration or pulmonary edema is suspected.

Pathogenesis Decreased serum pH increases toxicity by allowing more salicylate to diffuse into the CNS. Salicylates cause central respiratory drive stimulation, producing **hyperventilation and respiratory alkalosis** (the predominant clinical picture in adults). Salicylates also uncouple oxidative phosphorylation, resulting in **hyperthermia** and accumulation of lactate and organic acids, leading to a **metabolic acidosis** (the predominant presentation in children). **Confusion**, lethargy, seizures, and coma may be seen in severe cases. Gastric irritation causes vomiting that worsens **dehydration** and may lead to **hemorrhagic gastritis**.

Epidemiology **Children** are at risk for **accidental ingestion** of salicylate-containing products such as candy-flavored aspirin, oil of wintergreen (highly concentrated methylsalicylate), and Pepto-Bismol. The **elderly** are at risk for **chronic salicylate poisoning**.

Management **Intubate** obtunded patients to prevent aspiration. Give **activated charcoal** with a **cathartic**. Treat dehydration with **IV fluids**; replete **potassium** and restore electrolyte balance. Administer **sodium bicarbonate** to treat acidosis and **alkalinize urine** (alkaline urine "traps" salicylate in its ionic form and enhances elimination). **Hemodialysis** should be performed in cases of severe toxicity (progressive deterioration, coma, renal failure, salicylate level > 100 mg/dL, failure of medical treatment, or pulmonary edema). **Glucose** should be given IV even if hyperglycemia is not present because CNS glucose levels may be low in the face of normal serum glucose levels.

Complications Complications include **seizures**, coma, neurologic damage, and **arrhythmias** due to acidosis. In severe cases, platelet dysfunction and hypoprothrombinemia may occur. Noncardiogenic pulmonary edema may also occur.

MINICASE 69: HEAVY METALS TOXICITY

Multisystem (central and peripheral nervous system as well as GI, hematopoietic, renal, and cardiovascular system) toxicities due to heavy metals (most commonly lead, arsenic, and mercury), resulting from binding to sulfhydryl groups and disruption of enzymatic activity

- because physical complaints and findings (especially those involving the GI and nervous system) are numerous and nonspecific, a good occupational and environmental history is important
- urine, blood, and hair samples can be tested for levels
- CBC shows basophilic stippling with lead and arsenic toxicity
- x-rays detect lead lines in children, mercury poisoning may be associated with pulmonary emboli
- treat with supportive care, GI irrigation, and specific chelation therapy
- complications include encephalopathy and residual peripheral neurologic deficits

MINICASE 70: LEAD TOXICITY

Ingestion of gasoline, wall paint, or clay utensils

- presents with acute or subacute altered mental status, mental retardation in children, peripheral neuropathy, colicky abdominal pain, fatigue, ataxia, and purple lead lines on gums
- microcytic anemia with basophilic stippling, elevated blood lead levels, and elevated free erythrocyte protoporphyrin
- x-ray shows broad bands of increased density in long bones
- treat with EDTA, dimercaprol chelation, and avoidance of exposure

49 SALICYLATE TOXICITY

MINICASE 71: METHYLXANTHINE TOXICITY

Can be due to acute overdose or chronic toxicity

- presents with anxiety, vomiting, convulsions, hypertension, and tachycardia
- serum levels are elevated in acute disease but not in chronic toxicity
- treat with charcoal for acute overdose, benzodiazepines and beta-blockers to control autonomic hyperactivity
- complications include cardiac arrhythmias

MINICASE 72: SPIDER BITE—BROWN RECLUSE

The brown spider (2 to 3 cm in length with characteristic violin-shaped marking on its back) produces a cytotoxic and hemolytic venom that is capable of causing intense inflammation, tissue destruction, and hemolysis

- exposure commonly occurs in dark, wooded areas and presents with a localized stinging sensation, severe pain, pruritus, and systemic symptoms (rash, fever, chills, nausea, and vomiting)
- examination reveals a clear vesicle with an erythematous margin
- treat with debridement, cool compresses, antihistamines, dapsone
- complications include infection and skin necrosis (possibly requiring skin grafting), severe envenomation may result in hemolysis, DIC, renal failure, shock, and death

MINICASE 73: SPIDER BITE—WIDOW

Bites from brown, red, or black spiders (with an hourglass marking on the abdomen) result in toxin-mediated release of neurotransmitters, causing neurologic effects

- presents with pain followed within an hour by muscle cramping, nausea, vomiting, headache, and anxiety
- examination shows hypertension, tachycardia, diaphoresis, and muscle weakness
- CPK is often elevated
- treat with analgesics, benzodiazepines, antivenom
- complications include hypertensive emergency, respiratory difficulty, spontaneous abortion/preterm labor, rhabdomyolysis, and anaphylaxis